Sleep Surgery

Editor

STANLEY YUNG-CHUAN LIU

ATLAS OF THE ORAL AND MAXILLOFACIAL SURGERY CLINICS OF NORTH AMERICA

www.oralmaxsurgeryatlas.theclinics.com

Consulting Editor
RUI P. FERNANDES

March 2019 • Volume 27 • Number 1

ELSEVIER

1600 John F. Kennedy Boulevard • Suite 1800 • Philadelphia, Pennsylvania, 19103-2899
http://www.oralmaxsurgeryatlas.theclinics.com

ATLAS OF THE ORAL AND MAXILLOFACIAL SURGERY CLINICS OF NORTH AMERICA Volume 27, Number 1 March 2019 ISSN 1061-3315 ISBN-13: 978-0-323-65445-6

Editor: John Vassallo; j.vassallo@elsevier.com
Developmental Editor: Laura Fisher

Reprints. For copies of 100 or more of articles in this publication, please contact the Commercial Reprints Department, Elsevier Inc., 360 Park Avenue South, New York, NY 10010-1710. Tel.: 212-633-3874; Fax: 212-633-3820; E-mail: reprints@elsevier.com.

Atlas of the Oral and Maxillofacial Surgery Clinics of North America (ISSN 1061-3315) is published biannually by Elsevier, 360 Park Avenue South, New York, NY 10010-1710. Months of issue are March and September. Periodicals postage paid at New York, NY and additional mailing offices. Subscription prices are $455.00 for international individual, $396.00 for US individual, $416.00 for Canadian individual; $220.00 for international student and Canadian student, $100.00 for US student; $566.00 for international institution, $595.00 for Canadian institution, $461.00 for US institution. Foreign air speed delivery is included in all *Clinics* subscription prices. All prices are subject to change without notice. POSTMASTER: Send address changes to *Atlas of the Oral and Maxillofacial Surgery Clinics of North America*, Health Sciences Division, Subscription Customer Service, 3251 Riverport Lane, Maryland Heights, MO 63043. Tel: 1-800-654-2452 (U.S. and Canada); 314-447-8871 (outside U.S. and Canada). Fax: 314-417-8029. E-mail: journalscustomerservice-usa@elsevier.com (for print support); journalsonline support-usa@elsevier.com (for online support).

Atlas of the Oral and Maxillofacial Surgery Clinics of North America is covered in *MEDLINE/PubMed (Index Medicus)*.

Printed in the United States of America.

Contributors

CONSULTING EDITOR

RUI P. FERNANDES, MD, DMD, FACS, FRCS(Ed)
Clinical Professor and Chief, Division of Head and Neck Surgery, Departments of Oral and Maxillofacial Surgery, Neurosurgery, and Orthopaedic Surgery and Rehabilitation, University of Florida Health Science Center, University of Florida College of Medicine, Jacksonville, Florida, USA

EDITOR

STANLEY YUNG-CHUAN LIU, MD, DDS
Assistant Professor, Division of Sleep Surgery, Department of Otolaryngology, Co-director, Stanford Sleep Surgery Fellowship, Stanford University School of Medicine, Stanford, California, USA

AUTHORS

MICHAEL AWAD, MD, FRCSC
Division of Sleep Surgery, Department of Otolaryngology–Head and Neck Surgery, Stanford University School of Medicine, Stanford Hospital and Clinics, Stanford, California, USA

CARL BOUCHARD, DMD, MSc, FRCDC
Associate Professor of Oral and Maxillofacial Surgery, Service de chirurgie buccale et maxillo-faciale, CHU de Québec-Université Laval, Hôpital de l'Enfant-Jésus, Québec City, Québec, Canada

ROBSON CAPASSO, MD
Department of Otolaryngology–Head and Neck Surgery, Division of Sleep Surgery, Stanford Hospital and Clinics, Stanford, California, USA

ALLEN CHENG, DDS, MD, FACS
Head and Neck Surgical Associates, Medical Director, Oral/Head and Neck Cancer Program, Legacy Good Samaritan Cancer Center, Assistant Professor, Department of Oral and Maxillofacial Surgery, Oregon Health & Science University, Portland, Oregon, USA

STEPHEN T. CONNELLY, DDS, MD, PhD, FACS
Staff Surgeon, Oral and Maxillofacial Surgery Section, Department of Dental Service, San Francisco VA Health Care System, Associate Professor, Department of Oral and Maxillofacial Surgery, University of California, San Francisco, San Francisco, California, USA

GHALI E. GHALI, DDS, MD, FACS, FRCS(Ed)
Jack W. Gamble Professor, Chair, Department of Oral and Maxillofacial Surgery/Head and Neck Surgery, Louisiana State University Health Sciences Center – Shreveport, Shreveport, Louisiana, USA

CHRISTOPHER GOUVEIA, MD
Department of Otolaryngology–Head and Neck Surgery, Division of Sleep Surgery, Stanford Hospital and Clinics, Stanford, California, USA

CHRISTIAN GUILLEMINAULT, MD
Department of Psychiatry and Behavioral Sciences, Stanford Center for Sleep Sciences and Medicine, Stanford University School of Medicine, Stanford, California, USA

RISHI JAY GUPTA, DDS, MD, MBA
Chief, Oral and Maxillofacial Surgery Section, Department of Dental Service, San Francisco VA Health Care System, Assistant Professor, Department of Oral and Maxillofacial Surgery, University of California, San Francisco, San Francisco, California, USA; Assistant Professor, Department of Otolaryngology–Head and Neck Surgery, University of California, Davis, Sacramento, California, USA

JARED C. INMAN, MD
Associate Professor, Department of Otolaryngology–Head and Neck Surgery, Loma Linda University Health, Loma Linda, California, USA

SIMON JEAN, DMD
Oral and Maxillofacial Resident, Service de chirurgie buccale et maxillo-faciale, CHU de Québec-Université Laval, Hôpital de l'Enfant-Jésus, Québec City, Québec, Canada

DEEPAK KADEMANI, DMD, MD, FACS
Vice Chief of the Medical Staff, Medical Director, Department of Oral and Maxillofacial Surgery, Fellowship Director, Head and Neck Oncologic and Reconstructive Surgery, North Memorial Medical Center, Minneapolis, Minnesota, USA

UMAKANTH KATWA, MD
Department of Pediatrics, Division of Pulmonary and Sleep Medicine, Boston Children's Hospital, Instructor, Department of Pediatrics, Harvard Medical School, Boston, Massachusetts, USA

GI SOO LEE, MD, EdM
Department of Otolaryngology and Communication Enhancement, Boston Children's Hospital, Instructor, Department of Otolaryngology, Harvard Medical School, Boston, Massachusetts, USA

STANLEY YUNG-CHUAN LIU, MD, DDS
Assistant Professor, Division of Sleep Surgery, Department of Otolaryngology, Co-director, Stanford Sleep Surgery Fellowship, Stanford University School of Medicine, Stanford, California, USA

ANDREW T. MERAM, DDS, MD
Assistant Professor, Department of Oral and Maxillofacial Surgery/Head and Neck Surgery, Louisiana State University Health Sciences Center – Shreveport, Shreveport, Louisiana, USA

VLADIMIR NEKHENDZY, MD
Department of Anesthesia, Stanford Hospital and Clinics, Stanford, California, USA

KATINA NGUYEN, DDS
Resident, Department of Oral and Maxillofacial Surgery, Loma Linda University Health, Loma Linda, California, USA

TYLER S. OKLAND, MD
Department of Otolaryngology—Head and Neck Surgery, Stanford Hospital and Clinics, Stanford, California, USA

MÉLINDA PARIS, DMD, MSc, FRCDC
Oral and Maxillofacial Surgeon, Service de chirurgie buccale et maxillo-faciale, CHU de Québec-Université Laval, Hôpital de l'Enfant-Jésus, Québec City, Québec, Canada

ANTHONY POGREL, MD, DDS
Department of Oral and Maxillofacial Surgery, University of California, San Francisco, San Francisco, California, USA

CORY M. RESNICK, DMD, MD, FACS
Assistant Professor of Oral and Maxillofacial Surgery, Oral and Maxillofacial Surgeon, Department of Plastic and Oral Surgery, Boston Children's Hospital, Harvard School of Dental Medicine, Harvard Medical School, Boston, Massachusetts, USA

ROBERT WAYNE RILEY, MD, DDS
Clinical Professor of Otolaryngology, Stanford University School of Medicine, Stanford, California, USA

REBEKA SILVA, DMD, FACD
Staff Surgeon, Oral and Maxillofacial Surgery Section, Chief, Department of Dental Service, San Francisco VA Health Care System, Associate Professor, Department of Oral and Maxillofacial Surgery, University of California, San Francisco, San Francisco, California, USA

JAYINI S. THAKKER, DDS, MD
Assistant Professor, Department of Oral and Maxillofacial Surgery, Loma Linda University Health, Loma Linda, California, USA

CHRISTOPHER VUONG, MD
Resident, Department of Otolaryngology, Head and Neck Surgery, Loma Linda University Health, Loma Linda, California, USA

Contents

ATLAS OF THE ORAL AND MAXILLOFACIAL SURGERY CLINICS OF NORTH AMERICA

FORTHCOMING ISSUES

September 2019

Trauma Surgery
Robert A. Strauss and Alaaaldin Radwan, *Editors*

March 2020

Reconstruction of Facial Skin Defects
Anthony M. Bunnell, *Editor*

PREVIOUS ISSUES

September 2018

Sialendoscopy and Minimally Invasive Salivary Gland Surgery
Michael D. Turner and Maria J. Troulis, *Editors*

March 2018

Fat Grafting for Aesthetic Facial Surgery
Shahrokh C. Bagheri, Husain Ali Khan, and Behnam Bohluli, *Editors*

Preface

Sleep Surgery: From Reconstruction to Restoration and Re-education

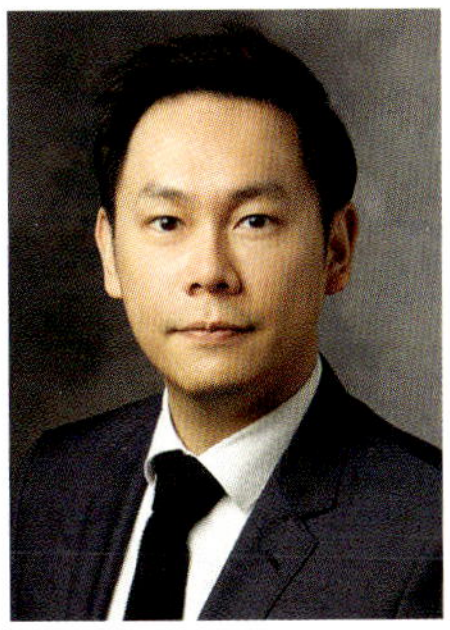

Stanley Yung-Chuan Liu, MD, DDS
Editor

I frequently show a slide that my mentors Dr Robert Riley and Dr Nelson Powell recount from 1979. The two sleep surgery pioneers were accomplished dental graduates of the University of California–San Francisco, who both then completed otolaryngology training at Stanford. They state:

The Sleep Center in 1979 was on the second story and the Otolaryngology Clinic was below. Dr Guilleminault and Dr Dement were interested in Bob Riley and I since we both had maxillofacial and dental experience. They were convinced that children and adults needed a more aggressive approach to OSAS than weight loss or a tracheotomy.

This was before the era of positive airway pressure therapy, and the vast knowledge about sleep and sleep apnea was yet to come. Dr Dement was the first physician-scientist to study sleep, and Dr Christian Guilleminault defined obstructive sleep apnea (OSA) in the modern era.

Sleep surgery has come a long way in just three decades. There is healthy discourse on indications, methodology, and efficacy. The role of surgery is not to replace, but to augment and complete the care a comprehensive sleep care team provides. It is not in a strict definition of surgical success where we rest our laurels, but in the patient's overall treatment success.

From that perspective, airway surgery for OSA is not merely reconstructive, it is also restorative in nature. Restoration of proper form allows re-education of healthy function.

I am thankful for the opportunity to gather oral and maxillofacial surgeons and otolaryngologists with maxillofacial expertise to share what we have learned. This is a mere start, and collectively, we will continue to restore sleep and dreams for our patients.

Stanley Yung-Chuan Liu, MD, DDS
Assistant Professor, Division of Sleep Surgery
Department of Otolaryngology
Co-director, Stanford Sleep Surgery Fellowship
Stanford University School of Medicine
801 Welch Road
Stanford, CA 94304, USA

E-mail address:
ycliu@stanford.edu

Atlas Oral Maxillofacial Surg Clin N Am 27 (2019) xi
1061-3315/19/© 2018 Published by Elsevier Inc.
https://doi.org/10.1016/j.cxom.2018.12.001

Sleep Surgery in the Era of Precision Medicine

Stanley Yung-Chuan Liu, MD, DDS [a,*], Robert Wayne Riley, MD, DDS [a], Anthony Pogrel, MD, DDS [b], Christian Guilleminault, MD [c]

KEYWORDS

• Obstructive sleep apnea • Sleep surgery • Maxillomandibular advancement • Transoral robotic surgery • Upper airway stimulation • Hypoglossal nerve • Genioglossus advancement • Palatopharyngoplasty

KEY POINTS

- Significant updates have been made to the original Stanford sleep surgery algorithm to reflect increased understanding of obstructive sleep apnea pathophysiology, patient phenotyping, and treatment outcome.
- Overall treatment success of the patient is more important than individual surgical success.
- The new algorithm focuses on precision in patient selection, procedural selection, and procedural accuracy.
- Positive airway pressure therapy plays a significant role in the surgical algorithm.
- Multilevel surgery or maxillomandibular advancement in combination with upper airway stimulation may achieve long-term cure.

How to approach a patient seeking surgery for obstructive sleep apnea?

A 52-year-old man with severe obstructive sleep apnea (OSA) and a history of septoplasty and uvulopalatopharyngoplasty (UPPP) seeks further care. Surgical options for him are not similar to those for a 22-year-old woman with mild OSA but presenting with equally debilitating daytime sleepiness and mood disturbance. What about a 64-year-old man with a history of nasal, palate, and maxillomandibular advancement (MMA) surgery 2 decades ago who now presents with moderate OSA? And what should be done with a patient with an apnea-hypopnea index (AHI) greater than 140 events per hour with normal body mass index (BMI), who is intolerant to continuous positive airway pressure (CPAP)?

Clearly, a surgical algorithm needs to be as patient-specific as possible, while incorporating all the established interventions in a systematic fashion.

Before presenting an updated sleep surgery algorithm based on 3 decades of experience at Stanford, several important points need to be made. They are the context through which the algorithm is conceived.

Disclosure Statement: None.

[a] Division of Sleep Surgery, Department of Otolaryngology, Stanford Sleep Surgery Fellowship, Stanford University School of Medicine, 801 Welch Road, Stanford, CA 94304, USA
[b] Department of Oral and Maxillofacial Surgery, University of California San Francisco, 533 Parnassus Ave, San Francisco, CA 94143, USA
[c] Department of Psychiatry and Behavioral Sciences, Stanford Center for Sleep Sciences and Medicine, Stanford University School of Medicine, 450 Broadway St, Redwood City, CA 94063, USA
* Corresponding author. 801 Welch Road, Stanford, CA 94025.
E-mail address: ycliu@stanford.edu

Why do we need an updated algorithm?

1. **Only one of the many OSA mechanisms is reliably addressed by surgical interventions : Airway critical closing pressure.**
   Interventions provided, including CPAP, affect airway critical closing pressure. There are other important mechanisms, including respiratory arousal threshold, muscle tone, and loop gain, which cannot be addressed directly by surgery.[1] Furthermore, loss of airway patency during sleep can be obstructive, mixed, or central in origin. Surgery mainly impacts obstructive apnea and hypopnea. Hence, a lot of humility must go into a surgeon's approach to OSA.
2. **The classic definition of "surgical success" is inadequate.**
   A frequently asked question is, "How successful is this surgery?" Literature has focused on surgical success, defined as AHI less than 20 events per hour or a decrease of more than half of the baseline AHI.[2] Is surgical success based on AHI adequate? First, the AHI needs to be interpreted with caution. The definition of hypopnea has changed several times from 1999 to 2012, and generally the definition has become more inclusive. In addition, there is inter-rater inconsistency in the interpretation of hypopnea.
   Second, it is increasingly difficult to obtain insurance approval for in-lab, attended polysomnography. Home sleep studies have become more common. The latter tend to present with lower AHI.
   Lastly, even the definition of surgical success has variation. Depending on the hypopnea and the surgical success criteria used, the same operation can be reported, with a success rate ranging from as low as 38.9% to as high as 91.7%.[3]
3. **Surgery can significantly decrease the burden of OSA, a chronic condition.**
   What patients need to be counseled on is that OSA and sleep-disordered breathing present on a continuum of

Atlas Oral Maxillofacial Surg Clin N Am 27 (2019) 1-5
1061-3315/19/
https://doi.org/10.1016/j.cxom.2018.11.012

severity and symptoms. It means that OSA can and does recur. It is a matter of how much and when. A relapse of 5 additional events per hour from AHI of 7 versus 70 does not have the same implications. This can be likened to playing field position in American football. The odds of scoring a touchdown is better when you are in the opposing team's red zone rather than your own.

4. **The patient chooses the procedure.**
Assuming the surgeon is able to offer or refer the full spectrum of contemporary sleep apnea surgery, it is still the patient who decides what procedure to undergo. A patient may be a logical candidate for MMA, but, if that is declined, it does not mean that surgeons cannot help with a combination of nasal and palate procedures followed by upper airway stimulation (UAS) of the hypoglossal nerve. A patient who is a good bariatric surgery candidate may decline that operation, but opt for nasal surgery to improve CPAP adherence. Sleep apnea surgery is elective; therefore, the surgeons' job is to maximize the treatment efficacy in every chosen option.

What is *precise* about the updated algorithm?

The updated algorithm adds precision in 3 areas.

1. Precision in patient selection with greater understanding of OSA pathophysiology and the use of diagnostic tools, such as drug-induced sedation (sleep) endoscopy (DISE) (Fig. 1).
2. Precision in introducing new procedures, such as UAS of the hypoglossal nerve or adult maxillary expansion (distraction osteogenesis maxillary expansion [DOME]), for previously unaddressed patient phenotypes (see Fig. 2).
3. Precision in performing established procedures with more accuracy and consistency. This includes tissue-sparing pharyngoplasty, transoral robotic surgery for lingual tonsillectomy, and virtual surgical planning (VSP) for skeletal procedures (see Fig. 2).

A brief word about the original Riley-Powell Stanford algorithm is interesting and important. Robert Riley and Nelson Powell obtained dental degrees from the University of California, San Francisco. They both obtained medical degrees, and Robert Riley also completed an oral and maxillofacial surgery residency at the University of California, Los Angeles. They became residents of otolaryngology at Stanford University. At this time, care for OSA patients entered a dynamic era. Stanford is the pioneering grounds of sleep medicine and research, with the world's first dedicated sleep clinic under Bill Dement. He first described rapid eye movement sleep.[4] Dr. Dement then recruited Christian Guilleminault, who first introduced sleep apnea.[5] Because the former Stanford otolaryngology and sleep medicine clinics were in the same building, the proximity and expert synergy among Guilleminault, Riley, and Powell produced the original Stanford sleep surgery algorithm. In the early 1990s, having the vision and capability to address both soft tissue and skeletal anatomic risk factors of OSA were defining for the field. Riley and Powell achieved high success and cure rates with patients going through phase 1 surgery—nasal, palate, and genioglossus advancement—followed by phase 2 surgery—MMA[6] (Fig. 1).

In contrast to the linear nature of the former Stanford algorithm, the new algorithm is on a continuum (Fig. 2). Specifics of each procedure are in other articles of this issue. This article serves as a formal introduction to the authors' current approach to sleep surgery patients.

How to optimize PAP or oral appliance therapy?

To begin, even if a patient is referred for surgery, a careful history about positive airway pressure (PAP) therapy needs to be undertaken. This is after having conducted a careful medical history as well. Patients with significant medical comorbidities or predominant central apnea are better treated with PAP therapy. A thorough nasal evaluation becomes critical, because treating nasal obstruction has been shown to decrease PAP pressure or increase adherence to PAP.[7,8] Septoplasty, inferior turbinate reduction, and/or nasal valve stabilization plays a significant role in acceptance and adherence to PAP. Nasal evaluation should not end with anterior rhinoscopy, because approximately 27% of patients who cannot tolerate

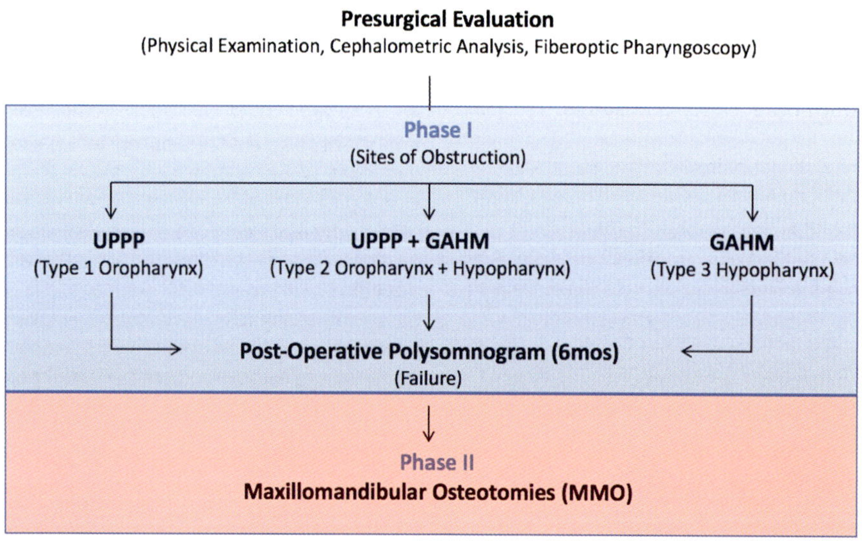

Fig. 1 Original Stanford sleep surgery algorithm. GAHM, genioglossus advancement with hyoid myotomy.

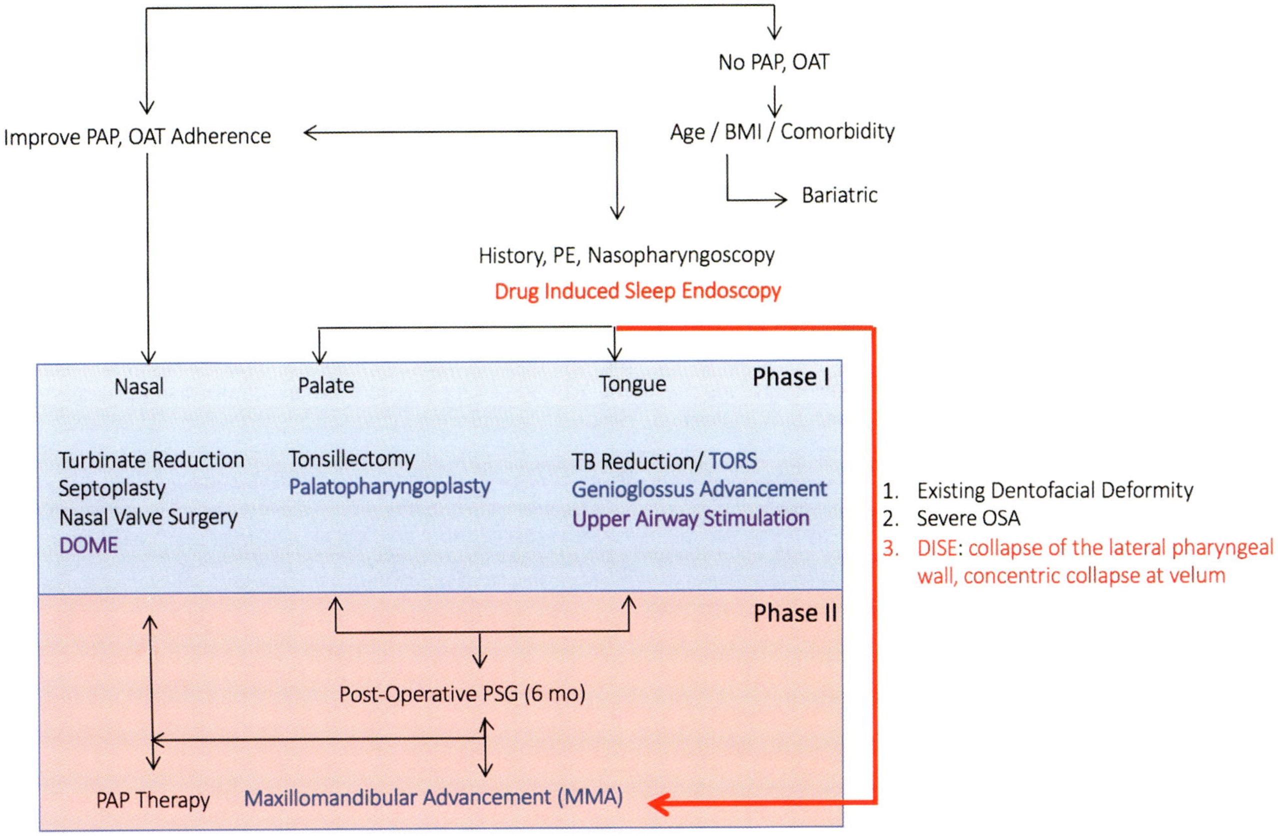

Fig. 2 Updated Stanford sleep surgery algorithm. PE, physical exam; PSG, polysomnography; TB, tongue base.

PAP present with posterior septal deviation that can be seen only by nasal endoscopy. This again is addressed with nasal surgery.

Less noticed as a key intervention for nasal obstruction is maxillary expansion. As evidenced in the pediatric literature, changing a high arched palate to a dome-shaped palate via rapid maxillary expansion treats nasal obstruction and OSA. The increase in nasal floor surface area decreases resistance through the internal nasal valve. Beyond improved nasal breathing, this also allows more intraoral volume for the tongue.[9–12] In 2015, Liu et al started performing adult maxillary expansion, described as DOME. DOME expands the nasal floor, increases the internal nasal valve angle, and decreases nasal resistance both objectively and subjectively in adults.[13]

Improving nasal breathing has an impact on not only PAP therapy but also oral appliance therapy (OAT). Although there are devices built to allow oral breathing, establishment of nasal breathing during sleep leads to more stable air flow and proper neurophysiologic effects on airway dilator muscles and improves sleep quality.[14,15]

For patients with elevated BMI, both medical and surgical management have significant roles.[16] Surgical intervention requires a period of maximal medical therapy; hence, referral to bariatric experts does not necessarily mean gastric bypass surgery. This can be helpful when counseling patients who are anxious about surgery as referrals are made.

Assuming patients have exhausted their PAP trial and evaluation, as described previously, and are willing to undergo surgery for OSA, the authors' sleep surgery algorithm continues as follows.

How to address the soft palate and tongue?

Although there are many different ways to perform tonsillectomy and palatopharyngoplasty, of greater importance is selecting patients who will do well with this procedure. This is well established by Friedman staging.[17] Contemporary palate surgery tends to be tissue-sparing, where the desired result is achieved by repositioning of dilator muscles rather than their resection.[18–20]

Surgery related to the tongue can be grouped into (1) genioglossus-based procedures, (2) tongue base and/or lingual tonsil removal, and (3) neurostimulation.

There are as many different ways to perform genioglossus advancement as there are to palatopharyngoplasty. It is more important to select the appropriate patient. Surgical success also increases when this is performed as part of a multilevel intervention.[13] Generally, to advance the genioglossus muscle, the osteotomy must capture the genial tubercle. For the suprahyoid muscles, the osteotomy must include the inferior border of mandible. The use of VSP with associated cutting guides has its place. As straightforward as this procedure can be, individual anatomic variations are accurately accounted for with VSP.[13]

There are both anterior and posterior approaches to resection of the tongue or lingual tonsillectomy as well as endoscopic and robot-assisted methods. With the advent of the single-port robot, which at the time of writing is not yet approved for use in OSA surgery, improved visualization and access may revolutionize transoral robotic surgery (TORS). TORS can readily access and address hypertrophic lingual tonsils, tongue fat, and the epiglottis.[21]

Although UAS of the hypoglossal nerve enacts on the tongue, the result is opening of the entire upper airway. Patient candidacy for the implant is based on DISE, where concentric collapse of the velum is a contraindication. AHI greater than 65 or predominantly central apnea are also contraindications. Only the hypoglossal nerve branches that protrude the tongue are included in the stimulation cuff, and the implant is tested prior to wound closure.[22–24] For patients showing concentric collapse of the velum or AHI greater than 65, additional procedures can be performed to mitigate the anatomic and physiologic contraindications. Isolated palate surgery, multilevel surgery, and MMA have all been performed prior to UAS by Stanley Liu to help patients meet selection criteria.[25]

When is skeletal surgery considered?

One of the most discussed questions is, "When can phase 2 (MMA) be performed before phase 1 procedures?"

The most straightforward MMA candidate is one with dentofacial deformity. This does mean, however, that a class 2 patient with OSA would undergo double jaw rather than mandibular advancement surgery alone. Maxillary advancement is a more significant contributor to MMA success.[26] This also means that a class 3 patient should not undergo the classic split-the-difference orthognathic planning, where the maxilla is advanced, and the mandible is setback. Most often, with counterclockwise rotation and advancement dictated by the maxilla, the mandible rotates and no setback is necessary. This is especially effective in patients with a high-angle class 3 dentofacial relationship.

Then there are class 1 patients with or without bimaxillary hypoplasia. This is often seen in patients with a history of extractions during orthodontic treatment. Historically, in creating functional occlusion via orthodontics alone, impact to the airway was not fully considered. This makes pediatric and adult maxillary expansion procedures critical. Although mandibular expansion may be needed in the pediatric population, adults with maxillary expansion often need only mandibular dental uprighting to re-establish proper occlusion. Regardless, the class 1 patient with or without bimaxillary hypoplasia can undergo MMA with airway-specific counterclockwise rotation in a surgery-first protocol. Only minimal perioperative orthodontic support is needed for optimal results.

An important additional selection criterion for MMA-first treatment planning resulted from observations during DISE. Classically, MMA is described as a form of hypopharyngeal surgery, mainly because the preoperative and postoperative lateral cephalometry or CT scan show a large increase in airway volume behind the tongue. Under DISE, however, it is clear that MMA significantly stabilizes the upper airway at the lateral pharyngeal wall and the velum (soft palate).[27,28] It readily reverses complete lateral pharyngeal wall collapse and concentric collapse of the velum. The discrepancy is easily explained. Maxillary advancement when performed properly stabilizes the tensor veli palatini, the palatoglossus, and the palatopharyngeus muscles. This cannot be observed via measurement of the radiographic airway space behind the soft palate in the midsagittal plane.

Therefore, assuming that the patient wishes to undergo MMA prior to other procedures, the indications include (1) preexisting dentofacial deformity; (2) AHI greater than 65 events per hour, where hypoglossal nerve stimulation is contraindicated and where multilevel soft tissue surgery may be inadequate; and (3) DISE findings of complete concentric collapse of the velum and lateral pharyngeal wall collapse.

At the time of this writing, the role of myofunctional therapy as an adjunct to the rehabilitation and re-education of upper airway muscles is under active investigation. If muscle remodeling is a significant reason for the success of MMA long-term, then both a faster return and maintenance of function may be augmented with properly selected upper airway exercises.[29]

What is the new definition of success?

3 patients scenarios reflect our response to this question:

1. A patient with high BMI declines bariatric surgery and elects for MMA. Even though the postoperative apnea index (AI) is zero (starting from 54), the postoperative AHI was still in the 50s (all hypopnea). This is a surgical failure by Sher's definition. He was able to use CPAP after MMA, however, where he was unable to do so before. He has been adherent to CPAP, and a year later returned with normalized BMI and greatly improved daytime symptoms.
2. A patient with a history of phase 1 and phase 2 operations 17 years ago returns with AHI slightly above 20. DISE shows no concentric collapse of the velum, and stable lateral pharyngeal wall. His tongue shows weak tone. He was offered UAS, which, when used, effectively brings his AHI to less than 5.
3. A 65-year-old man with normal BMI and lack of soft tissue redundancy presents with an AHI of 149 events per hour. MMA was performed, followed by UAS approximately 8 months later. His AHI was 17 events per hour after MMA and, after UAS, 4 events per hour.

In conclusion, the classic definitions of surgical success serve more as an academic guideline. The concept of treatment success is of greater importance and impact. Maximizing the efficacy of surgical interventions with proper patient selection and procedural expertise is critical, but success of any individual operation is not the end-goal. Treatment success of the patient results from the combination and continuum of medical and surgical interventions.

From this view, the new Stanford algorithm evolved from the fulfillment of best surgical practice and patient needs. Beyond the precision portrayed, it is the patient-centric nature of the new algorithm that defines its place for this dynamic era of sleep surgery.

References

1. Decker M, Yamauchi M, Strohl KP. Keep the airway open and let the brain sleep. Am J Respir Crit Care Med 2014;190(11):1207–9.
2. Sher AE. Update on upper airway surgery for obstructive sleep apnea. Curr Opin Pulm Med 1995;1(6):504–11.
3. Hobson JC, Robinson S, Antic NA, et al. What is "success" following surgery for obstructive sleep apnea? The effect of different polysomnographic scoring systems. Laryngoscope 2012;122(8): 1878–81.
4. Dement W, Kleitman N. Cyclic variations in EEG during sleep and their relation to eye movements, body motility, and dreaming. Electroencephalogr Clin Neurophysiol 1957;9(4):673–90.

5. Guilleminault C, Eldridge FL, Dement WC. Insomnia with sleep apnea: a new syndrome. Science 1973;181(4102):856–8.
6. Riley RW, Powell NB, Guilleminault C. Obstructive sleep apnea syndrome: a surgical protocol for dynamic upper airway reconstruction. J Oral Maxillofac Surg 1993;51(7):742–7 [discussion: 748–9].
7. Camacho M, Riaz M, Capasso R, et al. The effect of nasal surgery on continuous positive airway pressure device use and therapeutic treatment pressures: a systematic review and meta-analysis. Sleep 2015;38(2):279–86.
8. Powell NB, Zonato AI, Weaver EM, et al. Radiofrequency treatment of turbinate hypertrophy in subjects using continuous positive airway pressure: a randomized, double-blind, placebo-controlled clinical pilot trial. Laryngoscope 2001;111(10):1783–90.
9. Iwasaki T, Saitoh I, Takemoto Y, et al. Tongue posture improvement and pharyngeal airway enlargement as secondary effects of rapid maxillary expansion: a cone-beam computed tomography study. Am J Orthod Dentofacial Orthop 2013;143(2):235–45.
10. Iwasaki T, Saitoh I, Takemoto Y, et al. Improvement of nasal airway ventilation after rapid maxillary expansion evaluated with computational fluid dynamics. Am J Orthod Dentofacial Orthop 2012;141(3):269–78.
11. Iwasaki T, Takemoto Y, Inada E, et al. The effect of rapid maxillary expansion on pharyngeal airway pressure during inspiration evaluated using computational fluid dynamics. Int J Pediatr Otorhinolaryngol 2014;78(8):1258–64.
12. Machado-Junior AJ, Zancanella E, Crespo AN. Rapid maxillary expansion and obstructive sleep apnea: a review and meta-analysis. Med Oral Patol Oral Cir Bucal 2016;21(4):e465–9.
13. Liu SY, Guilleminault C, Huon LK, et al. Distraction osteogenesis maxillary expansion (DOME) for adult obstructive sleep apnea patients with high arched palate. Otolaryngol Head Neck Surg 2017; 157(2):345–8.
14. Ehsan Z, Ishman SL. Pediatric obstructive sleep apnea. Otolaryngol Clin North Am 2016;49(6):1449–64.
15. Ferguson KA, Ono T, Lowe AA, et al. A randomized crossover study of an oral appliance vs nasal-continuous positive airway pressure in the treatment of mild-moderate obstructive sleep apnea. Chest 1996;109(5):1269–75.
16. Wong AM, Barnes HN, Joosten SA, et al. The effect of surgical weight loss on obstructive sleep apnoea: a systematic review and meta-analysis. Sleep Med Rev 2018;42:85–99.
17. Friedman M, Ibrahim H, Bass L. Clinical staging for sleep-disordered breathing. Otolaryngol Head Neck Surg 2002;127(1):13–21.
18. Camacho M, Nesbitt NB, Lambert E, et al. Laser-assisted uvulopalatoplasty for obstructive sleep apnea: a systematic review and meta-analysis. Sleep 2017;40(3). https://doi.org/10.1093/sleep/zsx004.
19. Li HY, Lee LA. Relocation pharyngoplasty for obstructive sleep apnea. Laryngoscope 2009;119(12):2472–7.
20. Rashwan MS, Montevecchi F, Cammaroto G, et al. Evolution of soft palate surgery techniques for obstructive sleep apnea patients: a comparative study for single-level palatal surgeries. Clin Otolaryngol 2018;43(2):584–90.
21. Cammaroto G, Meccariello G, Costantini M, et al. Trans-oral robotic tongue reduction for OSA: does lingual anatomy influence the surgical outcome? J Clin Sleep Med 2018;14(8):1347–51.
22. Heiser C, Thaler E, Boon M, et al. Updates of operative techniques for upper airway stimulation. Laryngoscope 2016;126(Suppl 7): S12–6.
23. Strollo PJ Jr, Soose RJ, Maurer JT, et al. Upper-airway stimulation for obstructive sleep apnea. N Engl J Med 2014;370(2): 139–49.
24. Woodson BT, Strohl KP, Soose RJ, et al. Upper airway stimulation for obstructive sleep apnea: 5-year outcomes. Otolaryngol Head Neck Surg 2018;159(1):194–202.
25. Liu SY, Riley RW. Continuing the original stanford sleep surgery protocol from upper airway reconstruction to upper airway stimulation: our first successful case. J Oral Maxillofac Surg 2017;75(7): 1514–8.
26. Holty JE, Guilleminault C. Maxillomandibular advancement for the treatment of obstructive sleep apnea: a systematic review and meta-analysis. Sleep Med Rev 2010;14(5):287–97.
27. Liu SY, Huon LK, Iwasaki T, et al. Efficacy of maxillomandibular advancement examined with drug-induced sleep endoscopy and computational fluid dynamics airflow modeling. Otolaryngol Head Neck Surg 2016;154(1):189–95.
28. Liu SY, Huon LK, Powell NB, et al. Lateral pharyngeal wall tension after maxillomandibular advancement for obstructive sleep apnea is a marker for surgical success: observations from drug-induced sleep endoscopy. J Oral Maxillofac Surg 2015;73(8):1575–82.
29. Camacho M, Certal V, Abdullatif J, et al. Myofunctional therapy to treat obstructive sleep apnea: a systematic review and meta-analysis. Sleep 2015;38(5):669–75.

Drug-Induced Sleep Endoscopy

Michael Awad, MD, FRCSC [a,*], Tyler S. Okland, MD [b], Vladimir Nekhendzy, MD [c]

KEYWORDS

• OSA • Sleep endoscopy • Diagnostic sleep endoscopy • Drug-induced sleep endoscopy

KEY POINTS

- Obstructive sleep apnea is a heterogenous disorder characterized by a number of distinct phenotypes of upper airway collapse.
- Evaluating dynamic pharyngeal collapse in the sleeping patient is clinically challenging.
- Drug-induced sleep endoscopy is a safe, effective outpatient procedure for reliably assessing upper airway obstruction in the sleeping patient.
- Although numerous reporting methods exist for drug-induced sleep endoscopy findings, the VOTE (Velum, Oropharynx, Tongue base and Epiglottis) classification is the most widely used.

Video content accompanies this article at http://www.oralmaxsurgeryatlas.theclinics.com.

Introduction: nature of the problem

Obstructive sleep apnea (OSA) is a heterogeneous disorder represented by a wide spectrum of pharyngeal dysfunction. Modern surgical techniques are used to address the various clinical phenotypes. However, assessment of the site, extent, and severity of the obstructive event in the sleeping patient is a clinical challenge.

Early methods of assessment included Mueller's maneuver (forced inspiration against a closed glottis during awake endoscopy), lateral cephalometry, and computed tomography. However, these methods provided only static observations of the awake patient and could not identify dynamic, sleep-related obstructions. In 1991, Croft and Pringle[1] first proposed drug-induced sleep endoscopy (DISE) as a novel, outpatient technique for evaluating OSA. The technique described the use of medication-induced sleep in conjunction with fiberoptic endoscopy of the upper airway to develop a personalized airway approach for the sleep apneic patient. Before the introduction of DISE, a region-based approach to care was used by most sleep surgeons by categorizing patients according to the Fujita classification system.[2]

Owing to the need for a more targeted and clinically reliable means of characterizing patterns of upper airway obstruction, DISE has seen widespread adoption as one of the tools in clinical evaluation of the OSA patient and consideration of tailored surgical techniques. Although multiple classification systems have been proposed, the most widely adopted is the VOTE classification proposed by Kezirian and colleagues[3] in 2011. This classification is used to characterize DISE findings based on the specific structures (Velum, Oropharynx, Tongue base and Epiglottis) that most commonly contribute to upper airway obstruction. The VOTE classification has greatly improved the accuracy with which we can manage specific OSA phenotypes.

DISE is a necessary tool in the armamentarium of the sleep surgeon, allowing thorough and targeted evaluation of dynamic pharyngeal obstruction in the sleeping patient.

Surgical technique

Preoperative Planning

After undergoing thorough clinical assessment including a complete head and neck, and oral maxillofacial examination suitable candidates can be considered for DISE.

Required equipment

1. Recumbent patient bed
2. Distal chip-tip scope (author's preferred: Olympus ENF-VH High Definition Scope; Olympus, Tokyo, Japan)
3. Lidocaine jelly on a cotton-tipped applicator
4. Antifog solution

Preparation and patient positioning

The patient should be positioned supine and comfortable in a semidark and silent operating or endoscopy suite. In our practice, we do not provide oxygen supplementation to the patient during the procedure, in an attempt to correlate the endoscopy findings observed during patient's desaturation corresponding to the lowest nocturnal SpO_2. Standard patient monitoring includes

Disclosure: The authors have nothing to disclose.

[a] Division of Sleep Surgery, Department of Otolaryngology-Head and Neck Surgery, Stanford University School of Medicine, Stanford Hospital and Clinics, 801 Welch Road, Stanford, CA 95304, USA
[b] Department of Otolaryngology—Head and Neck Surgery, Stanford Hospital and Clinics, 801 Welch Road, Stanford, CA 95304, USA
[c] Department of Anesthesia, Stanford Hospital and Clinics, 801 Welch Road, Stanford, CA 95304, USA
* Corresponding author.
E-mail address: michaelawad@gmail.com

Atlas Oral Maxillofacial Surg Clin N Am 27 (2019) 7-10
1061-3315/19/
https://doi.org/10.1016/j.cxom.2018.11.010

pulse oximetry, electrocardiography, and noninvasive blood pressure measurement. Standard resuscitation equipment should be available. Lidocaine jelly applied to the nare can be applied for comfort before initiating endoscopy.

Anesthetic approach/sedation agent

Current data on sedative agents used in DISE remain limited, with limited study comparing obstruction to sleep staging with encephalography. Based on cardiac and pulmonary parameters, dexmedetomidine shows a more stable and potentially safer profile than propofol infusion.

Data from DISE patients induced with propofol have shown a greater degree of obstruction and desaturation observed than those induced with dexmedetomidine (Precedex). Propofol has been shown to demonstrate an oxygen nadir most representative of overnight polysomnography.[4] Pharmacologically, propofol also has a shorter half-life and quicker onset. However, the sedation with dexmedetomidine, a highly selective, centrally acting $\alpha 2$-adrenoreceptor agonist, affords a larger therapeutic window for respiratory depression/apnea compared with propofol.

A sedation with dexmedetomidine resembles natural sleep owing to a reduction of norepinephrine release by the locus coeruleus and subsequent release of γ-aminobutyric acid and galanin by the ventrolateral preoptic nucleus of the hypothalamus. A more gradual onset of dexmedetomidine-induced sedation/sleep also allows for ample time to observe dynamic airway behavior.

The prospective comparison studies on the use of different anesthetic techniques for DISE are lacking, and the choice of drug is often dictated by institutional preference. Yet, the paramount objective of allowing the surgeon to observe gradual onset of the upper airway collapse must be fulfilled with any technique. The sedation sequence is most commonly accomplished by administering an intravenous (IV) bolus of the selected drug (a loading dose), followed by an infusion.

The use of target-controlled infusions and other mathematical pharmacokinetic models, such as probability ramp control approach for administering propofol during DISE, has been shown to improve accuracy of achieving the required effect-site propofol concentration and reliability of the observational window for the obstructive events.[5–7] The predicted mean effect-site concentration for propofol during DISE ranges between 2.0 and 4.8 μg/mL, with the loss of upper airway tone occurring at 2.94 ± 0.97 μg/mL, and upper airway obstruction at 4.2 ± 1.3 μg/mL.[8]

Because target-controlled infusions are not currently available in the United States, in our practice we rely on manual-controlled propofol infusions. Our typical approach involves administering the background infusion of IV propofol 150 to 180 μg/kg/min with the superimposed small IV propofol boluses 0.1 to 0.2 mg/kg every 30 seconds. In our experience, this sequence assures a reliable and gradual upper airway collapse within 5 to 7 minutes.

For a dexmedetomidine DISE sequence, we administer dexmedetomidine IV bolus 1.5 μg/kg over 10 minutes, followed by infusion of 1.5 μg/kg/h. A reliable induction of sleep and upper airway collapse is observed in the vast majority of patients within 15 minutes, with occasional top-up dexmedetomidine rapid IV boluses 0.25 μg/kg required after the administration of the loading dose had been completed.

Surgical procedure

As sedation is administered, the surgeon places the distal chip-tip scope into the nare identifying the side with least obstruction. The scope is passed through the middle meatus, above the inferior turbinate, and directly inferior to the middle turbinate and passed posteriorly until the nasopharynx is reached. From this position, the scope is positioned in a rostral view (facing toward the larynx) to best visualize the velum as sedation is infused.

After observation at the level of the velum is complete and the degree of obstruction is noted, the scope is passed distally to observe the airway at the level of the oropharynx. Subsequently, the scope is passed to observe the tongue base and epiglottis. Observed findings are recorded in a table as described in Fig. 1.

Additional measures that are annotated include:

A. Lowest O_2 saturation
B. Improvement of desaturation with jaw thrust
C. Improvement of desaturation with mouth closure

Care should be taken by the endoscopist to note additional structures of interest, such as mass lesions of the upper aerodigestive tract, enlarged adenoids, or laryngeal pathologies such as subglottic stenosis (Figs. 2 and 3, Videos 1–3).

Potential complications

Although complications from DISE are rare, care should be taken to ensure optimal patient safety, particularly in the obese patient and those with severe OSA who are likely to demonstrate lower pulmonary reserve and an increased propensity for rapid oxygen desaturation. The specific end point of anesthetic administration in DISE is airway obstruction without intentional oversedation necessitating airway intervention. The average practicing anesthesiologist will have limited experience with this form of gradual propofol titration and so expected administration protocols and safety measures should be clearly outlined by the endoscopy team before initiation. Risks include allergic reaction and, although commonly communicated, recent

STRUCTURE	DEGREE OF OBSTRUCTION[a]	CONFIGURATION[c]		
		A-P	LATERAL	CONCENTRIC
Velum				
Oropharynx lateral walls[b]				
Tongue Base				
Epiglottis				

Fig. 1 The VOTE classification. A-P, anteroposterior. [a] Degree of obstruction is graded for each structure: 0, no obstruction (no vibration); 1, partial obstruction (vibration); 2, complete obstruction (collapse); X, not visualized. [b] Oropharynx obstruction can be distinguished as related solely to the tonsils or including the lateral walls, with or without a tonsillar component. [c] Configuration is noted for structures with degree of obstruction greater than 0. (*From* Kezirian EJ, Hohenhorst W, de Vries N. Drug-induced sleep endoscopy: the VOTE classification. Eur Arch Otorhinolaryngol 2011;268(8):1233–6; with permission.)

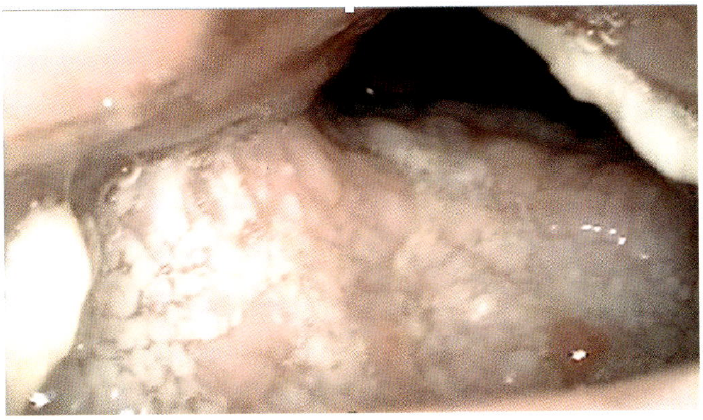

Fig. 2 Isolated partial (grade: 1) tongue base collapse.

studies indicate patients with soy, glycerol, or egg do not have an increased risk of allergic reaction with propofol administration.[9–11] Second, epistaxis may occur secondary to placement of the endoscope and care should be taken to avoid undue trauma to the nasal mucosa during endoscopy.

Bradycardia and hypotension have been demonstrated in association with both propofol and dexmedetomidine, further highlighting the importance of continued monitoring and preparedness for managing these rare but potentially acute complications.[12]

Finally, and most of concern, is oversedation leading to airway obstruction. Sedation, whether with propofol or dexmedetomidine, should be administered slowly under continuous monitoring in every case and in a facility with capacity and equipment to rapidly intubate should complete obstruction not responsive to other airway measures such as bag-mask, jaw thrust, nasal trumpets, and other airway adjuncts fail.

Immediate postoperative care

DISE is performed as an outpatient procedure with no need for overnight observation in most circumstances. Patients should be monitored in a recovery setting with 1:1 nursing after emergence from anesthesia and can be discharged the same day with assistance. Care should be taken to inform patients not to drive after undergoing anesthesia.

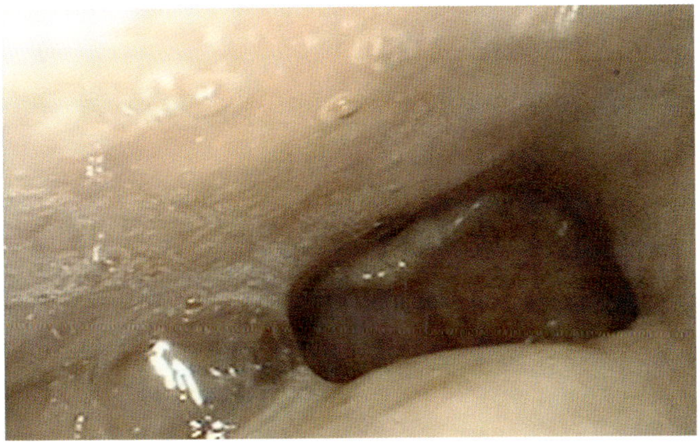

Fig. 3 Isolated complete (grade: 2) anteroposterior epiglottis collapse.

Pearls and pitfalls

The relatability of DISE to naturally induced sleep has been discussed in the literature at length. Propofol-induced sleep induces a lower minimum O_2 saturation (SaO_2) than natural sleep. Propofol-induced sleep also results in a significant change in sleep architecture with an increase in N3 (deep or slow-wave) sleep. Finally, there is also a marked inability to observe rapid eye movement sleep during propofol sedation, a period during which OSA is known to worsen in severity.[13]

Clinical results in the literature

DISE is used to identify unique OSA phenotypes and thereby tailor treatment strategies. Koutsourelakis and colleagues[14] found complete circumferential collapse of the velum was an important independent predictor of upper airway surgery failure. Complete lateral pharyngeal wall collapse has been demonstrated to show a strong association with disease severity, thus indicating a need for more aggressive treatment strategies in this group of patients.[15] Furthermore, DISE has been used to demonstrate improved stability of the lateral pharyngeal walls in patients who undergo maxillomandibular advancement procedures. The degree of lateral wall stability has been directly correlated with improvements in the apnea-hypopnea index.[16]

Beyond surgical intervention, DISE is also used to determine the impact of jaw thrust maneuvers on obstruction and help predict the likelihood of success with oral appliance therapy. A retrospective review by Huntley and colleagues[13] demonstrated patients with increased airway dimensions at the level of the velum and/or oropharynx with a jaw thrust during DISE benefitted most from oral appliance therapy. Similarly, DISE has been shown to be a useful adjunct in titrating continuous positive airway pressure therapy in treatment-resistant patients.[17,18]

Today, the most widely applicable use of DISE in the United States is determination of candidacy for upper airway stimulation. The absence of palatal complete circumferential collapse is an indication for upper airway stimulation implantation and has been demonstrated to predict therapeutic success.[19] In other words, an anteroposterior pattern of collapse at the level of velum is favorable for patient selection in upper airway stimulation.

Of note, increased age also seems to impact DISE findings. A case series by Zhao and colleagues[20] demonstrated age is an independent risk factor for increased apnea-hypopnea index, combined levels of obstruction, and complete anteroposterior velum collapse pattern during DISE.

Systematic evaluation of the upper airway with DISE remains somewhat heterogenous. A recent systematic review by Amos and colleagues[21] reported no consensus reporting method for DISE findings, although the VOTE classification remains the most commonly used at 38.6%.

Summary

DISE is a safe and clinically useful tool for targeting surgical therapy, irrespective of the choice of sedation. It can also aid in the optimization of medical therapy, including oral appliances, positional devices, and continuous positive airway pressure. Beyond medical therapy, DISE is used to determine candidacy for upper airway stimulation and demonstrate disease severity in at-risk patients. The value of the procedure continues to evolve and expand, with newer applications such as titrating treatment failure after upper airway stimulation being described.

Supplementary data

Supplementary data related to this article can be found online at https://doi.org/10.1016/j.cxom.2018.11.010.

References

1. Croft CB, Pringle M. Sleep nasendoscopy: a technique of assessment in snoring and obstructive sleep apnoea. Clin Otolaryngol Allied Sci 1991;16(5):504–9.
2. DNF F, Fujita S, Ikematsu T, et al. Snoring and obstructive sleep apnea. 1987:101–28.
3. Kezirian EJ, Hohenhorst W, de Vries N. Drug-induced sleep endoscopy: the VOTE classification. Eur Arch Otorhinolaryngol 2011;268(8):1233–6.
4. Viana A, Zhao C, Rosa T, et al. The effect of sedating agents on drug-induced sleep endoscopy findings. Laryngoscope 2018;158: 1259.
5. Atkins JH, Mandel JE, Rosanova G. Safety and efficacy of drug-induced sleep endoscopy using a probability ramp propofol infusion system in patients with severe obstructive sleep apnea. Anesth Analg 2014;119(4):805–10.
6. De Vito A, Agnoletti V, Zani G, et al. The importance of drug-induced sedation endoscopy (D.I.S.E.) techniques in surgical decision making: conventional versus target controlled infusion techniques—a prospective randomized controlled study and a retrospective surgical outcomes analysis. Eur Arch Otorhinolaryngol 2017;274(5):2307–17.
7. Mandel JE, Sarraf E. The variability of response to propofol is reduced when a clinical observation is incorporated in the control: a simulation study. Anesth Analg 2012;114(6):1221–9.
8. Borek RC, Thaler ER, Kim C, et al. Quantitative airway analysis during drug-induced sleep endoscopy for evaluation of sleep apnea. Laryngoscope 2012;122(11):2592–9.
9. Asserhøj LL, Mosbech H, Krøigaard M, et al. No evidence for contraindications to the use of propofol in adults allergic to egg, soy or peanut†. Br J Anaesth 2016;116(1):77–82.
10. Harper NJN. Propofol and food allergy. Br J Anaesth 2016;116(1): 11–3.
11. Tashkandi J. My patient is allergic to eggs, can I use propofol? A case report and review. Saudi J Anaesth 2010;4(3):207–8.
12. Cho JS, Soh S, Kim EJ, et al. Comparison of three sedation regimens for drug-induced sleep endoscopy. Sleep Breath 2015;19(2):711–7.
13. Huntley C, Cooper J, Stiles M, et al. Predicting Success of Oral Appliance Therapy in Treating Obstructive Sleep Apnea Using Drug-Induced Sleep Endoscopy. J Clin Sleep Med 2018;14(8):1333–7.
14. Koutsourelakis I, Safiruddin F, Ravesloot M, et al. Surgery for obstructive sleep apnea: sleep endoscopy determinants of outcome. Laryngoscope 2012;122(11):2587–91.
15. Lan M-C, Liu SYC, Lan M-Y, et al. Lateral pharyngeal wall collapse associated with hypoxemia in obstructive sleep apnea. Laryngoscope 2015;125(10):2408–12.
16. Liu SY-C, Huon L-K, Powell NB, et al. Lateral pharyngeal wall tension after maxillomandibular advancement for obstructive sleep apnea is a marker for surgical success: observations from drug-induced sleep endoscopy. J Oral Maxillofac Surg 2015;73(8): 1575–82.
17. Lan M-C, Hsu Y-B, Lan M-Y, et al. The predictive value of drug-induced sleep endoscopy for CPAP titration in OSA patients. Sleep Breath 2017;4(1):53–6.
18. Torre C, Liu SY, Kushida CA, et al. Impact of continuous positive airway pressure in patients with obstructive sleep apnea during drug-induced sleep endoscopy. Clin Otolaryngol 2017;42(6): 1218–23.
19. Vanderveken OM, Maurer JT, Hohenhorst W, et al. Evaluation of drug-induced sleep endoscopy as a patient selection tool for implanted upper airway stimulation for obstructive sleep apnea. J Clin Sleep Med 2013;9(5):433–8.
20. Zhao C, Viana A, Ma Y, et al. The effect of aging on drug-induced sleep endoscopy findings. Laryngoscope 2018;7(pt 2):1311.
21. Amos JM, Durr ML, Nardone HC, et al. Systematic review of drug-induced sleep endoscopy scoring systems. Otolaryngol Head Neck Surg 2018;158(2):240–8.

Further reading

Chang ET, Certal V, Song SA, et al. Dexmedetomidine versus propofol during drug-induced sleep endoscopy and sedation: a systematic review. Sleep Breath 2017;21(3):727–35.

Nasal Surgery for Sleep-Disordered Breathing

Jayini S. Thakker, DDS, MD [a,*], Christopher Vuong, MD [b], Katina Nguyen, DDS [a], Jared C. Inman, MD [b]

KEYWORDS

• Obstructive sleep apnea • Nasal examination • Site of obstruction • Nasal surgery • Nasal obstruction

KEY POINTS

- Nasal obstruction, like other obstructive sleep breathing disorders, is multifactorial with many areas of potential anatomic obstructions. This article reviews the role of nasal obstruction in these complicated patients.
- The nasal examination should follow a structured approach in describing and quantifying areas of nasal obstruction before planning surgery for patients with obstructive sleep apnea.
- Identifying the area of nasal obstruction and its related surgical options are reviewed with a focus on the physical examination and anatomic considerations.

Introduction

Nasal obstruction accounts for half of airway resistance and may contribute to the development of sleep-disordered breathing, including upper airway resistance syndrome and obstructive sleep apnea (OSA) in certain individuals.[1] When this is identified in a patient with sleep-disordered breathing, surgery can be offered, but it is important that the techniques used be tailored to the specific sites of obstruction identified.

Identifying the site of nasal obstruction

Examination of the nasal cavity should proceed in a systematic and reproducible manner to improve communication among physicians and guide surgical treatment. Rhinoscopy typically involves assessment pre- and postapplication of a topical decongestant to observe the effects of inflammation on nasal obstruction. Partial nasal obstruction is far more common than complete obstruction.

Presence of a deviated septum is extremely common. In some studies, a deviated septum is even more prevalent than a nondeviated septum.[2] The anatomic location of the septal deformity is important in determining if an individual will have nasal obstruction symptoms, if any. For example, even small deflections of the anterior septum can cause significant obstruction because of the septum's location within the nasal valve, whereas posterior deflections generally need to be much larger to similar obstructive symptoms.[3]

Disclosure: The authors have nothing to disclose.

[a] Department of Oral and Maxillofacial Surgery, Loma Linda University Health, 11092 Anderson Street, Room 3305, Loma Linda, CA 92354, USA

[b] Department of Otolaryngology, Head and Neck Surgery, Loma Linda University Health, 11234 Anderson Street, Loma Linda, CA 92354, USA

* Corresponding author. 11092 Anderson Street, Suite3305, Loma Linda, CA 92354.

E-mail address: jthakker@llu.edu

Classifying the position of septal deflection therefore plays an important role in guiding the type of surgery. The most commonly accepted measurements of the septum involve qualitative and quantitative measurements. Quantitatively, septal deviation can be graded as 0% to 25% deflection, 26% to 50% deflection, 51% to 75% deflection, and 76% to 100% deflection from the midline to the lateral nasal wall.[4] Qualitatively, septal deviation may be described as either cephalocaudal or anteroposterior and further divided into C-shaped, reverse C-shaped, S-shaped, or reverse S-shaped.[4,5]

Similar to septal deflections, inferior turbinate hypertrophy is clinically important because of its involvement at the lateral boundary of the internal nasal valve. Hypertrophy can be classified as bony, soft tissue, or mixed, which may direct the type of surgery indicated, that is, turbinectomy for bony hypertrophy versus soft tissue submucous resection. Inferior turbinate size can be reported based on the degree of obstruction caused by the head of the inferior turbinate relative to the total airway space. This is graded as 0% to 25%, 26% to 50%, 51% to 75%, and 76% to 100%.[6]

Surgical technique

In the following narrative, the authors outline common techniques/maneuvers in a traditional patient with nasal obstruction resulting from static middle septal deviation and enlarged inferior turbinates (Fig. 1). For more complicated cases, it may be prudent to refer to an experienced specialist for surgery. Although the traditional closed septoplasty technique is best suited for middle septal deflections, dorsal or caudal deflections may be best suited for open rhinoplasty with grafts and techniques beyond the scope of this article.

Anesthesia and analgesia

Before any surgical steps, inspection of the nasal cavity should proceed before decongestion to assess potential areas of

Atlas Oral Maxillofacial Surg Clin N Am 27 (2019) 11–16

https://doi.org/10.1016/j.cxom.2018.11.009

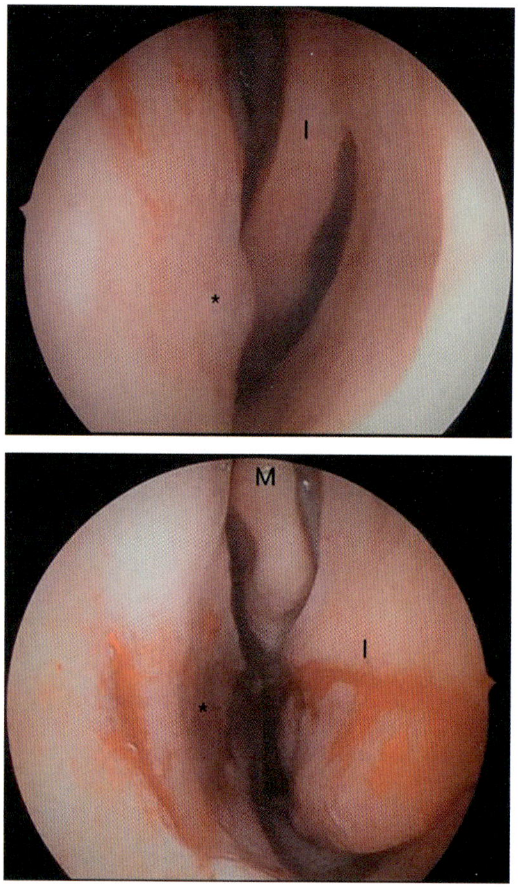

Fig. 1 Preoperative view of septal spur/obstruction (*top*) and postoperative view (*bottom*). (*Asterisk*) Septal spur/obstruction; (I) inferior turbinate; (M) middle turbinate.

obstruction. Decongestion is achieved with either 4% cocaine or more commonly oxymetazoline on pledgets that are placed into the nasal cavity for vasoconstriction. This reduces bleeding, creates space for instrumentation, and also allows improved visualization of the septum. Minimizing bleeding is paramount for visualization during nasal surgery, and for this reason the patient is also placed in reverse Trendelenburg position.

In addition to vasoconstriction, injection of 1% lidocaine with 1:100000 epinephrine into the septal mucoperichondrial plane also aids in hydrodissection before elevation. Injection begins posteriorly to prevent bleeding anteriorly, which would otherwise distort visualization of the posterior septum during injection. Typically a 25 or 27 gauge needle is advanced with the bevel parallel to the septum until slight resistance is met taking care not to go through to the contralateral side. Injection will be met with some resistance from the septum impeding flow of anesthetic, at which point the needle is withdrawn slightly until the anesthetic is able to be easily injected with almost instant transient blanching of the mucosa. This is repeated in multiple areas along the superior-inferior plane while moving anteriorly and injecting the incision site. The contralateral membrane should also be injected as well as the area around the maxillary crest. After the injection is performed, waiting at least 15 to 20 minutes will ensure maximum vasoconstriction, which is why it is a common practice to inject immediately after intubation.

Incision

Incision location is variable and generally reliant on surgeon preference. Traditionally, for the right-handed surgeon, he or she stands at the right of the patient and creates the incision in the left nare. However, many surgeons prefer to make the incision on the side with the largest spur or most prominent deflection. Of note, mucosal incisions are placed anterior to the start of the deflection or obstruction. There are 3 types of incisions—Killian, hemitransfixion, and full transfixion—each with specific advantages and disadvantages. A Killian incision (Fig. 2) is made approximately 1 to 2 cm posterior to the caudal septal margin within the respiratory epithelium and is useful for middle septal deviations. Caudal septal deviations are more difficult to access and easier to create tears in the flap due to delicate nature of the anterior respiratory mucosa.

A hemitransfixion (see Fig. 2) or transfixion incision made at the caudal border of the cartilaginous septum allows access to caudal deflections. In contrast to the Killian, the incision is created within the squamous epithelium of the vestibule in the membranous septum. Conversion to a full-transfixion incision is easily accomplished by incising completely through to the opposite membrane; however, this may reduce nasal tip support and is not usually necessary. Other approaches such as the transcolumellar incisions used in open rhinoplasty are beyond the scope of this article and will not be discussed.

Elevating the mucoperichondrial flap

A hemitransfixion incision outline is created by using the nasal speculum to push the membranous septum toward the contralateral nare to expose the caudal septal edge and create tension before making the incision. A No. 15 blade is used to incise through mucosa and perichondrium to the cartilage layer, which has the appearance of a white and rough surface.

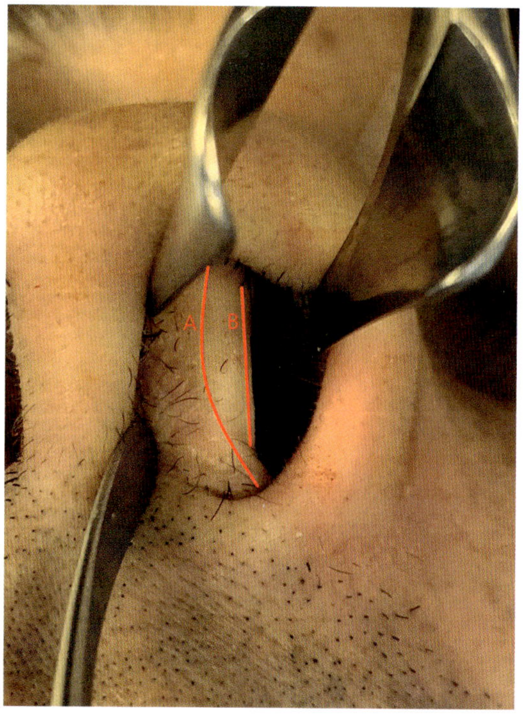

Fig. 2 Types of closed septoplasty incisions. (A) Hemitransfixion/transfixion; (B) Killian.

This incision may be extended to the nasal floor, which is helpful for inferior septal deviations. The dissection proceeds in the subperichondrial layer to minimize bleeding and creates a more durable flap, which decreases the likelihood of perforation. This may be achieved by "scraping" the perichondrium off the cartilage with a sharp edge such as the Cottle elevator or No. 15 blade. Once in the subperichondrial plane, further elevation of the flap is typically initiated with the Cottle elevator and then continued with the dull side of the Cottle or a freer (Fig. 3). It is important to raise the flap atraumatically by "sweeping" the instrument in the direction of the least resistance and continuing to enlarge the pocket, making sure the instrument is in contact with the septum at all times. This can be accomplished with direct visualization using a narrow speculum or more commonly by feel and tracking the plane of least resistance. Of note, areas of fracture or severe deflections often have trapping, duplication, or adherence of planes and more sharp dissection under direct visualization is necessary to prevent rents. Rents are often created due to forceful instrumentation in the anterior to posterior direction or from angling the instrument off the septum, which may occur during concave portions of the septum. If a hole is created, one should reduce propagation of the rent by avoiding strong suction at the edge of the rent. Two tunnels should be elevated superiorly and inferiorly to the rent and connected, which may require scraping off adherent mucosa with the Cottle elevator.

As one moves from anterior to posterior, longer nasal specula are inserted between the mucoperichondrial flap and cartilage to improve visibility posteriorly as one continues elevating the flap. One can minimize tearing of the flap by elevating superiorly and inferiorly as far as possible to reduce tethering of the flap, thereby reducing tension. A common mistake is to not elevate far enough inferiorly, which may cause a surgeon to overlook maxillary crest deviations or the septum that has shifted off the crest, causing inferior airway obstruction. Elevating subperiosteally over the maxillary crest may require using a Cottle elevator or No. 15 blade to sharply dissect through the dense fibrous attachments of the maxillary crest. Dissection then continues past the bony-cartilaginous junction to gain access to any posterior bony deflection or spur. At this time, the Cottle elevator may be used to separate the bony and cartilaginous septal segments to prepare for removal of cartilage once the opposing mucoperichondrial flap is elevated.

During elevation, one should take special care when encountering septal spurs, which are typically tightly adherent to the thinned overlying mucosa. Elevation may be achieved by creating 2 pockets or tunnels superiorly and inferiorly of the septal spur to reduce tension, then gently connecting the 2 tunnels to release any adhesions. For tightly adherent mucosa, sharper spade end of the Cottle elevator may be used to carefully scrape and release the mucosa. Creating tears is sometimes unavoidable but further propagation should be avoided and extra care should be made to prevent bilateral tears.

Removing the obstruction

After the membrane is elevated on one side, a contralateral flap is elevated by first creating a transcartilaginous incision (Fig. 4) 1 to 2 mm anterior to the most caudal aspect of the septal deviation with a Cottle elevator or D knife. Preservation of the "L strut" is important to prevent saddle-nosed deformities or compromising tip support by ensuring a 1-cm dorsal and caudal aspect of the septum. One should only remove the obstructing portion of the septum because excessive removal can lead to floppy septums and subsequent perforation.

The Cottle elevator is then used to initiate the opposing mucoperichondrial flap and elevation is continued with a freer in similar fashion with a superior-inferior "sweeping" fashion to elevate past the obstruction (Fig. 5). If needed, a small window may be created by taking a small piece of cartilage with a takahashi or nonbiting forceps. After ensuring flaps are elevated bilaterally on either side of the obstruction, the cartilage piece is then excised. There are multiple ways to excise the obstructing piece. If using a swivel knife, the knife is seated on the most dorsal border of the planned incision and moved in the anterior-posterior direction until bone is met. The knife is then brought inferiorly to the maxillary crest and carried parallel to the floor in an anterior direction until the cartilage is completely excised. If using a D knife or scalpel, a superior incision is made to the boney-cartilaginous junction and then a Cottle or freer may be used to detach the posterior border and along the maxillary crest. A nonbiting forceps such as a takahashi is then used in a rotary fashion to break off the remaining pieces of attachment. Utmost care to prevent forceful detachment of the dorsal septum to the ethmoid plate should be used to prevent cribriform destabilization and

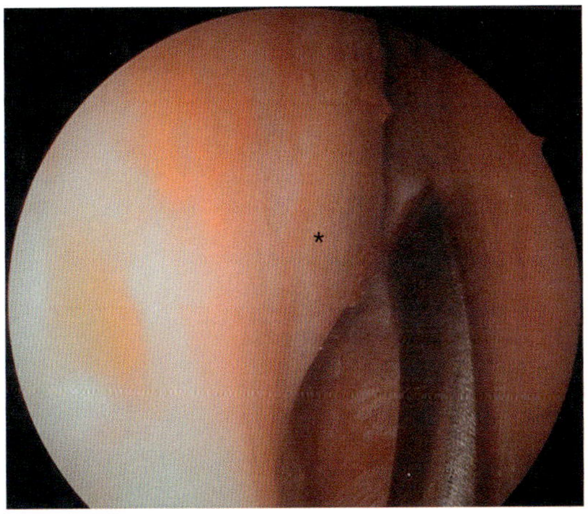

Fig. 3 Elevation of mucoperichondrial flap over septal spur/obstruction. (*Asterisk*) Septal spur/obstruction.

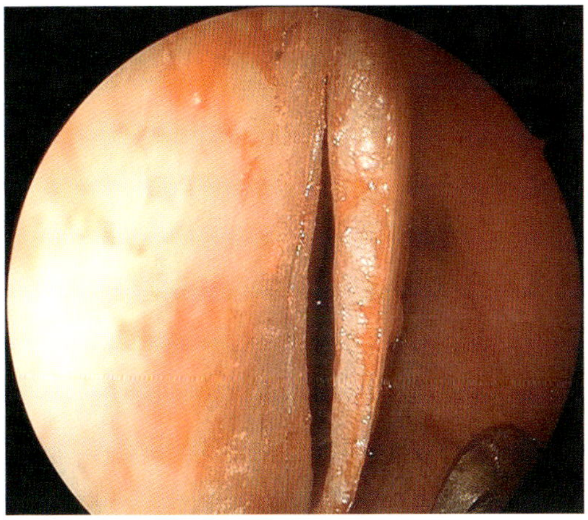

Fig. 4 Transcartilaginous incision.

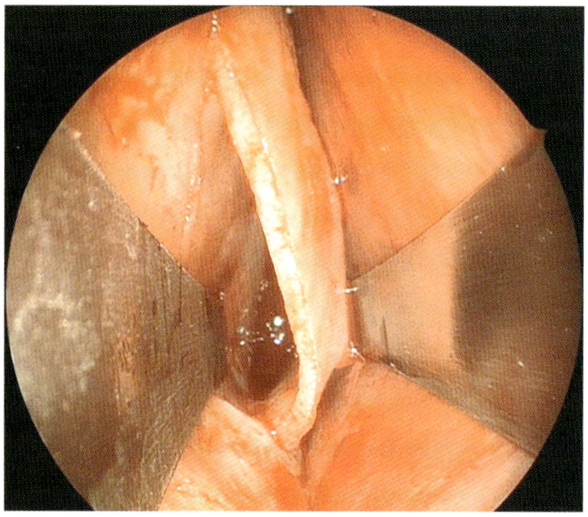

Fig. 5 Bilateral elevation of mucoperichondrial flaps.

cerebrospinal fluid (CSF) leak. This is prevented by completely releasing the obstructing cartilage piece from its dorsal attachments before removal and then using cutting instruments such as Jansen-Middleton to remove further dorsal segments.

Ensuring proper elevation of bilateral mucoperichondrial flaps is also important to reduce massive tears when pulling out pieces of cartilage that are still adherent to mucosa. If there is any resistance during cartilage removal, attempt to identify and remove any adherent points before trying again. Removing cartilage in one piece is preferred if grafting material is planned later during the operation.

After removing the obstructing cartilage and any residual pieces, there is improved visualization of the posterior boney septum, which may have been blocked by obstructing cartilage segments (Fig. 6). Further elevation of bilateral subperiosteal flaps may be raised, and boney deviations may be removed with Jansen-Middleton forceps. Straight pieces should be contoured and placed back in the mucoperichondrial plane once the surgery is complete if they do not need to be sacrificed.

Deviations frequently occur when the quadrilateral cartilage is shifted off the crest, leading to nasal floor obstruction. Removal of the maxillary crest may be achieved with a 4-mm osteotome or a V-chisel taking care to not completely transect the crest in order to avoid injury to the nasopalatine nerve or greater palatine artery. In cases where cartilage is subluxed off the maxillary crest or bowed to one side, a "swinging door" may be created by incising the inferior aspect of the cartilage off the maxillary crest. This superiorly based mobile segment is then relocated to the maxillary crest and the most anterior-inferior aspect is sutured to periosteum of maxillary spine with 5′0 polydioxanone. If there is still bowing of this segment, excess cartilage may be trimmed inferiorly before securing with suture. If most of the obstruction is limited to one side, a conservative approach may be to shave the offending portion parallel to the crest with a 2 mm osteotome or No. 15 blade. Scoring of cartilage without resection, with or without grafting, is another option that involves using a knife to weaken the concave aspect of bowed defects, which subsequently release the septum back midline.

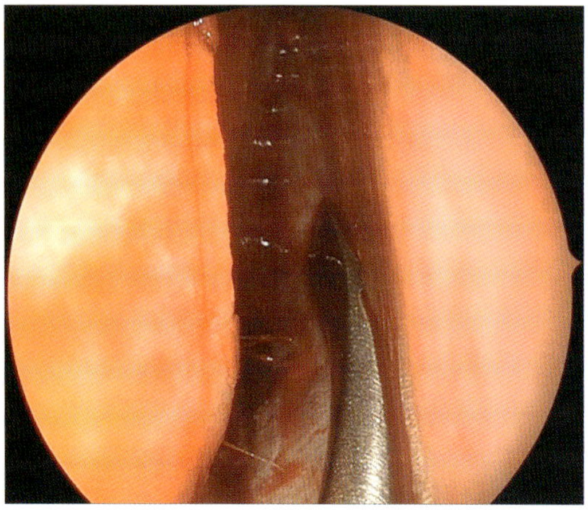

Fig. 6 View after obstructing septal spur was removed.

Closure

After removing the obstructing cartilage and bone, the mucoperichondrial flaps are coapted together to prevent hematoma collection by using either a quilting suture or silastic splints, or both. In general, packing has fallen out of favor for patient comfort and lack of proven utility, with the exception of bleeding that cannot be isolated and stopped. A continuous quilting suture is made with a 5′0 chromic on a Keith or curved needle with an anchoring knot at the end to prevent pulling the suture through the mucosa. Suturing begins posteriorly and moves anteriorly as one passes the needle back and forth from one side of the septum to the other along various levels. Alternatively, bilateral Doyle splints may be used by itself or in conjunction with quilting suture and is inserted flat against the septum and secured transeptally through the membranous septum with a 4′0 prolene. Before insertion of doyle splints, the incision site is closed with 5′0 chromic and any large rents may be repaired with 5′0 chromic or incorporated into the quilting suture with bilateral rents often necessitating a biological mesh.

Endoscopic approach

Endoscopic septoplasty is primarily useful in patients with mid- to posterior deflections, which are difficult to visualize through the standard closed septoplasty approach. The incision and initiation of the mucoperichondrial flap is typically carried out in the traditional way with or without an endoscope. After initial elevation of flaps, the endoscope is placed under the flap and dissection is continued with endoscopic guidance. During this process, a freer with suction capabilities (suction freer) is helpful to aid visualization. After elevation of the flap past the posterior obstructing segment, the remainder of the septoplasty is the same as the traditional approach in regard to the transcartilaginous incision, elevation of the contralateral mucoperichondrial flap, and excision of the obstructing segment under endoscopic guidance. Another advantage of an endoscopic approach is that the incision can be placed much more posterior directly in front of the deflection and the anterior tissues can remain undissected.

Inferior turbinate reduction

There have been many alternatively described techniques for inferior turbinate reduction, including radiofrequency, laser, and cryosurgery. A large study comparing several of these modalities found submucosal resection with outfracture to have the best outcome at 6 years and is currently the preferred technique with slight modification.[7,8]

Inferior turbinate reduction is performed before the septoplasty portion of the procedure and begins with injection of 1% lidocaine with 1:100,000 epinephrine under direct visualization using a nasal speculum or endoscope. Using a scalpel or leading edge of the microdebrider, a stab incision is made at the head of the turbinate, and the soft tissue is elevated off the underlying bone with a freer, Cottle, or microdebrider. After elevating a pocket, the soft tissue is then removed using a microdebrider or Blakesley. The microdebrider's oscillating blade is directed away from the turbinate bone and controlled resection proceeds at a low speed taking care to preserve the overlying mucosa. Soft tissue reduction should be concentrated near the anterior two-thirds of the inferior turbinate, which causes most obstruction. Similarly, a cost-saving measure would be to use the Blakesley forceps to reduce soft tissue along with the anterior one-half to two-thirds of the turbinate bone if needed. Our standard procedure also includes controlled electrocautery of the submucosal tissue at the head of the inferior turbinate for tissue reduction while taking care to preserve mucosa to prevent sloughing postoperatively. An extended bovie tip may also be used for more posterior submucosal resection if needed.

Outfracture is then performed by placing a freer in the inferior meatus and fracturing the turbinate upward and medially. A Boies-Goldman or Freer elevator is then placed on the superior and medial surface of the turbinate and is outfractured laterally and inferiorly due to the angle at which the inferior turbinate attaches to the lateral wall. If the turbinate bone is medially displaced or enlarged and not responding to outfracture, it can also be removed anteriorly while preserving the mucosa.

Complications

Early complications

As with traditional cosmetic septorhinoplasty, surgical manipulation of the nasal septum, lateral cartilages, and turbinates for the purpose of sleep surgery can result in many of the same complications. These may include intraoperative or early complications, as well as late or delayed complications weeks to months after surgery.

The most common intraoperative complication is excessive hemorrhage, most often from septal vascular plexuses. Hemorrhage can typically be prevented or controlled with topical vasoconstrictors (cocaine, phenylephrine) or injection of local anesthetic with epinephrine. If these measures fail, one can use conservative electrocautery and apply pressure until bleeding settles. These interventions will typically suffice for anterior bleeds, but posterior bleeds may necessitate posterior packing to tamponade the bleeding, or even selective arterial embolization, which is an exceedingly rare necessity.

Early infections are rare and may result from use of foreign materials such as Gore-Tex (polytetrafluoroethylene); these must be recognized and treated immediately to prevent serious sequelae, such as cavernous sinus thrombosis. CSF leak is another rare occurrence and can be recognized as a clear watery nasal discharge, which may increase with valsalva. This can result from high resection of the perpendicular plate of the ethmoid bone, resulting in violation of the cribriform plate, or even aggressive manipulation of nasal bones without adequate osteotomy mobilization. However, this is not a maneuver that would typically be done when addressing isolated nasal obstruction, unless concomitant esthetic issues were being addressed.

If a hematoma develops postoperatively, it must be recognized and evacuated immediately; it will typically present as a painful, ecchymotic mass on the septum and may also result in mild fever. Septal hematoma should be drained emergently to avoid septal pressure necrosis and potential loss of mucosa and cartilage, which can result in septal perforation and may even compromise the architectural support of the nose.

Late complications

Septal perforation can also be a late/delayed complication of septal surgery. This is most often due to bilateral mucosal tears that overlap. A perforation can also arise in patients who use intranasal cocaine recreationally or in patients who may have developed a septal hematoma or infection after surgery compromising perfusion to the septum. Infection after routine septoplasty is rare and is typically seen when foreign materials are placed or when hematomas are not adequately treated.

Loss of tip support and/or saddle nose deformity may result from aggressive resection of cartilage. Preservation of a 1 to 1.5 mm L-strut along the dorsal and caudal septal cartilage will prevent this complication. Internal nasal valve collapse may be a result of scarring along the incision site or due to over-resection of upper or lower lateral cartilages. The treatment for this is revision surgery, with removal of scar tissue and placement of spreader grafts.

Other complications

In addition, when manipulating the airway in a patient with sleep-disordered breathing, there is always the potential to transiently exacerbate the duration and severity of apneas due to nasal obstruction in the immediate postoperative period, as a result of mucosal congestion, as well as nasal packings, and residual blood, which may take weeks to be completely evacuated. In rare cases, the nasal obstruction may actually even worsen long after surgery. For instance, improper technique may result in iatrogenic collapse of cartilaginous structures. Or if meticulous wound closure and tissue management is not ensured, synechiae may develop, resulting in worsening of obstruction. These are infrequent occurrences but must be recognized when they do present postoperatively.

Because of the limited range of surgical techniques described in this article (septoplasty, select grafting techniques, and inferior turbinate reduction), the authors have only listed complications related to those procedures they outlined. However, one may come across unique complications, when using techniques to address various other sites of nasal obstruction.

Discussion

The role of nasal surgery in OSA treatment remains elusive, with most published cohorts demonstrating minimal to no improvement in the apnea-hypopnea index and respiratory disturbance index. Typically only mild OSA and snoring are treated effectively with nasal surgery; however, patients have subjective improvements in quality of life parameters such as sleep quality, daytime sleepiness, snoring, and overall quality of life compared with their preoperative state. The other benefit from nasal surgery is increased continuous positive airway pressure (CPAP) compliance among patients due to more comfortable CPAP pressures and the ability to switch to more tolerable nasal appliances once obstruction has been relieved.[9,10]

Part of the reason many studies do not show objective improvement in OSA with nasal surgery is because they do not take into consideration the multilevel theories of obstruction. Nasal obstruction, similar to the multilevel approach of sleep surgery, has specific subsites that need to be identified and addressed in order to effectively treat sleep-disordered breathing.

Summary

Although there is little experimental data regarding the benefit of nasal surgery in patients with OSA, nasal surgery may be effective in treating mild OSA and snoring and improving CPAP compliance. In addition, accurate diagnosis and patient selection are imperative for directing surgical approaches and ensuring predictable outcomes.

References

1. Verse T, Pirsig W. Impact of impaired nasal breathing on sleep-disordered breathing. Sleep Breath 2003;7:63–74.
2. Gray LP. Deviated nasal septum.Incidence and etiology. Ann OtolRhinolLaryngol Suppl 1978;87(3 Pt 3 Suppl 50):3–20.
3. Becker DG, Ransom E, Guy C, et al. Surgical treatment of nasal obstruction in rhinoplasty. AesthetSurg J 2010;30(3):347–78 [quiz: 379–80].
4. Rohrich RJ, Gunter JP, Deuber MA, et al. The deviated nose: optimizing results using a simplified classification and algorithmic approach. PlastReconstr Surg 2002;110(6):1509–23 [discussion: 1524–5].
5. Camacho M, Zaghi S, Certal V, et al. Predictors of nasal obstruction: quantification and assessment using multiple grading scales. PlastSurg Int 2016;2016:6945297.
6. Camacho M, Zaghi S, Certal V, et al. Inferior turbinate classification system, grades 1 to 4: development and validation study. Laryngoscope 2015;125(2):296–302.
7. Passali D, Passali FM, Damiani V, et al. Treatment of inferior turbinate hypertrophy: a randomized clinical trial. Ann OtolRhinolLaryngol 2003;112(8):683–8.
8. Mickelson SA. Nasal surgery for obstructive sleep apnea syndrome. OtolaryngolClin North Am 2016;49(6):1373–81 [review].
9. Zonato AI, Bittencourt LR, Martinho FL, et al. Upper airway surgery: the effect on nasal continuous positive airway pressure titration on obstructive sleep apnea patients. Eur Arch Otorhinolaryngol 2006;263:481–6.
10. Friedman M, Tanyeri H, Lim JW, et al. Effect of improved nasal breathing on obstructive sleep apnea. Otolaryngol Head Neck Surg 2000;122:71–4.

Tonsillectomy and Pharyngoplasty

Tissue-Preserving Techniques

Michael Awad, MD, FRCSC [a,*], Christopher Gouveia, MD [a], Robson Capasso, MD [a], Stanley Yung-Chuan Liu, MD, DDS [b]

KEYWORDS

• OSA • Pharyngoplasty • Palatopharyngoplasty • Palatal expansion

KEY POINTS

- The airway of obstructive sleep apnea (OSA) patients has been shown to be smaller in the lateral dimension and retropalatal region.
- Palatopharyngoplasty can be performed alone or in conjunction with other OSA surgeries.
- In appropriately selected patients, palate procedures are highly effective at enlarging the retropalatal space and stabilizing the lateral pharyngeal walls.
- Tissue-preserving techniques are preferred for avoiding complications and maximizing efficacy.

Introduction

The geometry and caliber of the upper airway of patients with obstructive sleep apnea (OSA) have been shown to differ from that of healthy controls. The airway of patients with OSA has been shown to be smaller, primarily in the lateral dimension and the retropalatal region.[1] Often referred to as the workhorse of sleep apnea surgery, palatopharyngoplasty (PPP) is performed alone or in conjunction with other OSA surgeries. The procedure, which encompasses several technical variations, including uvulopalatopharyngoplasty (UPPP), sphincter pharyngoplasty, and expansion pharyngoplasty (discussed later), enlarges the retropalatal airway via the excision of tonsil tissue (if present), trimming and reorientation of the anterior and posterior tonsillar pillars, and excision of a portion of the uvula and soft palate.

The likely origin of modern palatopharyngoplasty techniques dates back to the 1950s when Schwartz used resection of paramedian soft palate triangles on either side of the uvula in the treatment of snoring.[2] However, the procedure most reminiscent of the palatopharyngoplasty performed today was later described by Ikematsu in Japan in 1964 after seeing a female patient who was divorced due to her loud snoring. Several iterations of the procedure have since been introduced, with Simmons and colleagues[3] advocating for excision of the uvula versus the traditional uvular repositioning technique seen with Fujita's approach.[4]

Traditionally, UPPP has been and continues to be the most commonly performed of pharyngeal procedures. Historically, the Fujita classification has been used to assess the upper airway. Fujita's classification describes 3 patterns of upper airway collapse, essentially divided into upper (type I), lower (type II), and combined (type III) pharyngeal collapse.

Surgical technique: preoperative planning

After initial evaluation, including thorough history and physical examination, including fibreoptic nasendoscopy, all patients undergoing PPP for OSA should have documented evidence of OSA or snoring. During the head and neck examination, particular care should be paid to tonsil size, palate redundancy, uvular length, and tongue base position as well as general body habitus and calculation of body mass index. Close attention to these clinical features is critical in ensuring appropriately selected patients and thus optimal results, with patient selection being shown to be the primary factor in determining the wide variety in surgical success seen in the literature.[5] Performance of Muller's maneuver can also aid in determining the level or levels of airway obstruction in each specific clinical scenario.

Surgical approaches

Transitioning from a uvular excision technique, in 1996 Powell and colleagues[6] introduced the uvulopalatal flap (UPF) technique, which involves repositioning the uvula and posterior soft palate anteriorly. With this technique, the palatal muscles are preserved, which reduces the risk of velopharyngeal insufficiency, a feared consequence of overresection of the soft palate. In contrast to traditional UPPP, where incisions are made along the interior surface of the palate and the lateral pharyngeal well, UPF incisions are made on the oral surface of the soft palate, which has been demonstrated to reduce

Disclosure Statement: The authors have nothing to disclose.

[a] Division of Sleep Surgery, Department of Otolaryngology-Head and Neck Surgery, Stanford University School of Medicine, Stanford Hospital and Clinics, 801 Welch Road, Stanford, CA 95304, USA
[b] Division of Sleep Surgery, Department of Otolaryngology, Stanford Sleep Surgery Fellowship, Stanford University School of Medicine, 801 Welch Road, Stanford, CA 94304, USA
* Corresponding author.
E-mail address: Michaelawad@gmail.com

Atlas Oral Maxillofacial Surg Clin N Am 27 (2019) 17-22

https://doi.org/10.1016/j.cxom.2018.11.005

circumferential scar, thus reducing postoperative pain as well as the risk of bleeding.[6]

In contrast to PPP and UPF, transpalatal advancement pharyngoplasty, described in the early 1990s, stabilizes the upper airway by altering bone and soft tissue attachments of the posterior maxilla rather than radical modification of the palatal soft tissue and musculature. This technique makes use of a shorter palatal flap and greater palate mobilization than traditional PPP, with an osteotomy used to advance the palate that has soft tissue attached to the osteotomized bone fragment.

Interestingly, lateral pharyngeal wall narrowing has been shown to be the sole oropharyngeal finding on examination that predisposes to Obstructive Sleep Apnea Hypopnea Syndrome in men.[7] As a result of this finding, lateral pharyngoplasty was proposed in which the tonsils are removed in standard fashion. Following tonsillectomy, the palatoglossus and palatopharyngeus muscles are identified, and using an operative microscope, the superior pharyngeal constrictor muscle is elevated and sectioned in a cranial-caudal direction. This results in 2 muscle flaps: first, a medially based flap, and second, a laterally based flap, which is sutured anteriorly to the ipsilateral palatoglossus muscle with a series of 3 stitches. Finally, a transverse incision on the oral surface of the soft palate is made extending laterally from the base of the uvula extending superiorly to create a laterally based palatine flap. In order to close the tonsillar fossa, the palatopharyngeus muscle is sectioned in a transverse fashion creating a superior flap that is sutured with a Z-plasty along with the palatine flap to cover the superior portion of the tonsillar fossa. The inferior palatopharyngeus muscle flap is used to suture closed the inferior aspect of the tonsillar fossa.[8] Although the procedure has shown promising results, patients frequently complain of postoperative dysphagia.

Another variation on PPP, expansion sphincter pharyngoplasty, was originally borne from the treatment of velopharyngeal incompetence in cleft palate patients by creation of a dynamic muscle sphincter. The procedure begins with tonsillectomy, followed by rotation of the palatopharyngeus muscle. The inferior portion of the palatopharyngeus is transversely sectioned, rotated superolaterally, and fixed with a figure-of-8 suture. An incision is then made on the anterior pillar arches to identify the palatoglossus muscle fibers, such that the rotated palatopharyngeus muscle can be fixed to the palatoglossus fibers. Next, a partial uvulectomy is performed and the anterior and posterior pillars are sutured together, opposing these 2 surfaces.[9]

Surgical technique

The patient is first positioned supine on the operating table and undergoes induction and oral intubation with an oral RAE endotracheal tube. The procedure can be performed in a seated or standing position. After induction and intubation, a mouth gag, in the form of a Boyle-Davis or a Tonsil A-Frame, is used to prop the mouth open with care taken to ensure the tongue and endotracheal tube are fixed in a midline position without obscuring either of the tonsillar beds (Fig. 1).

Tonsillectomy is performed in the standard fashion (Figs. 2–3). The authors prefer the use of monopolar cautery to identify an extracapsular plane and facilitate removal of the tonsils from superior to inferior. Diligent care is taken to ensure meticulous hemostasis after removal of the tonsils with a combination of oxymetazoline-soaked pledgets, bipolar cautery, and/or suction cautery.

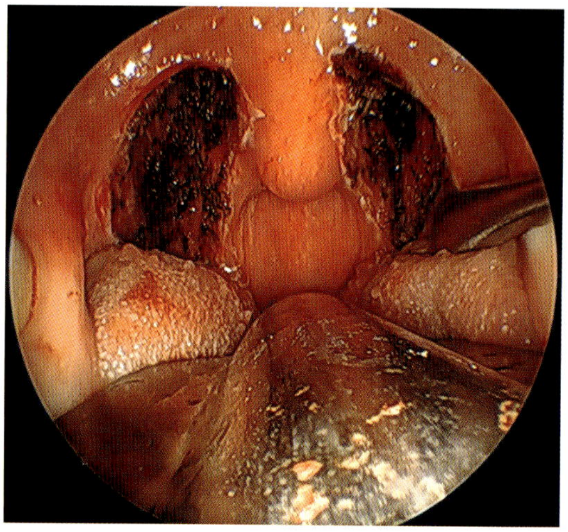

Fig. 1 Tonsillectomy is performed in the standard fashion. Monopolar cautery is our preferred technique.

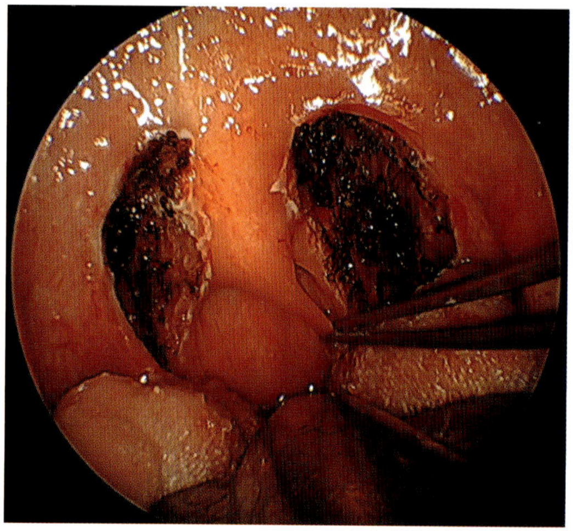

Fig. 2 After removal of the tonsils, the uvula is grasped with a toothed-forceps and trimmed.

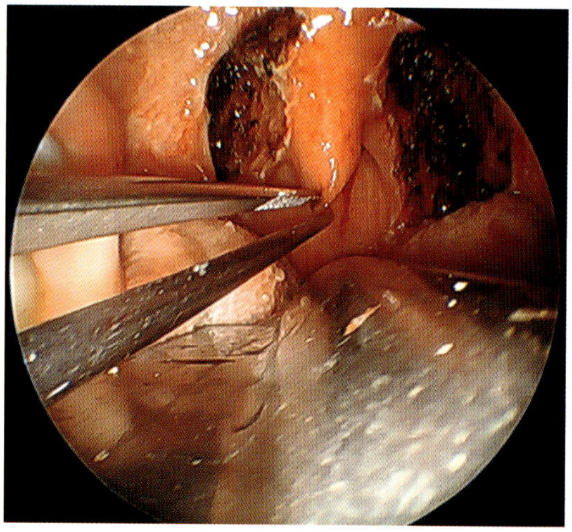

Fig. 3 The uvula is trimmed to prevent elongated and redundant mucosa.

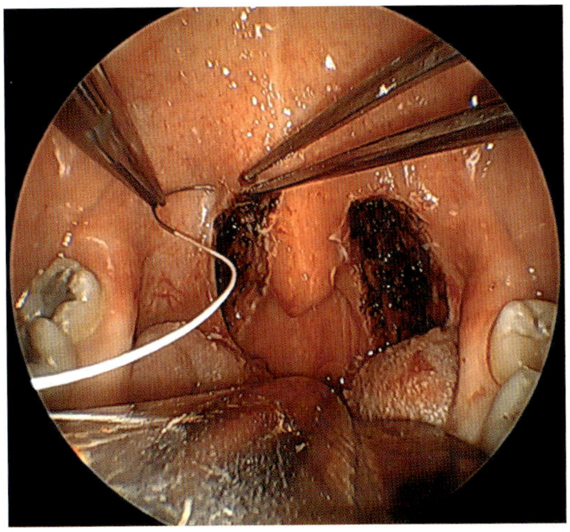

Fig. 4 Following uvulectomy, attention is turned to the palatopharnygoplasty portion of the procedure.

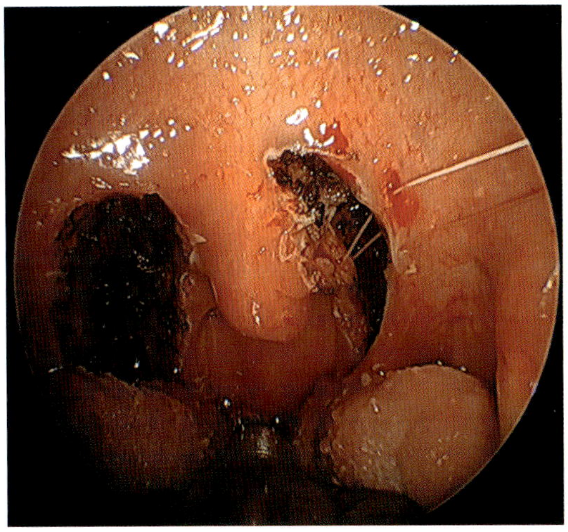

Fig. 6 These 45 degree sutures oppose the tonsillar pillars while encompassing the tensor veil palatini muscle.

After removal of the tonsils, the uvula is grasped with a non-toothed forceps and trimmed to a length of 1 cm with the use of a monopolar cautery. The uvula should be trimmed in a V-shape to facilitate velopharyngeal closure rather than a straight-line resection. Use of monopolar cautery facilitates further volume reduction of the uvula due to thermal-assisted fibrosis and also aids in achieving hemostasis and reducing postoperative bleeding.

Following uvulectomy, attention is turned to the pharyngoplasty portion of the procedure (Figs. 4–7). With the use of a 3-0 Vicryl suture, a series of 3 horizontal mattress sutures are placed from anterior to posterior pillar and then back through the anterior pillar. These are tied down to an appropriate tension in series. Depending on the individual length of the pillar, 3 to 4 horizontal mattress sutures can be placed in each tonsillar fossa (Fig. 8).

Appearance of right tonsillar fossa after completion of one side of the pharyngoplasty procedure is described above. Three 3-0 Vicryl sutures have been placed facilitating significant lateral pharyngeal wall expansion (Fig. 9).

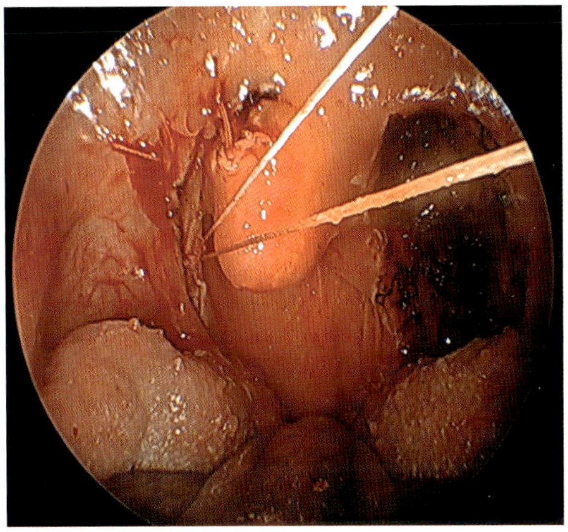

Fig. 7 A second 3–0 absorbable mattress suture is used to suspend the palatopharyngeus muscle creating expansion of the lateral pharyngeal wall.

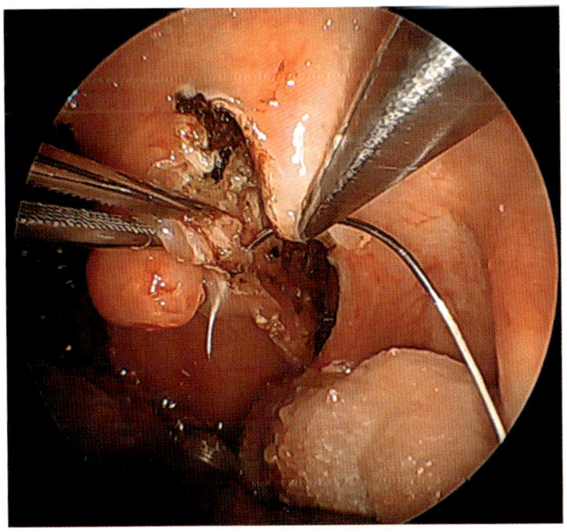

Fig. 5 3–0 absorbable mattress sutures (Vicryl pop-offs) are used in a 45-degree plane to suspend and oppose the anterior and posterior pillars.

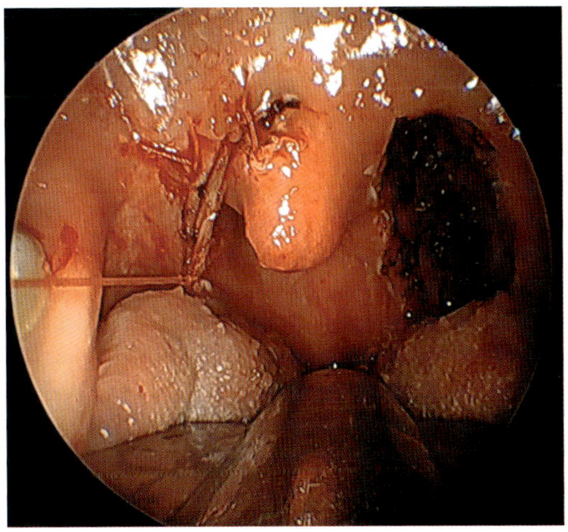

Fig. 8 Depending on the length and suspension achieved a second horizontal mattress suture can be placed to further suspend the lateral pharyngeal wall.

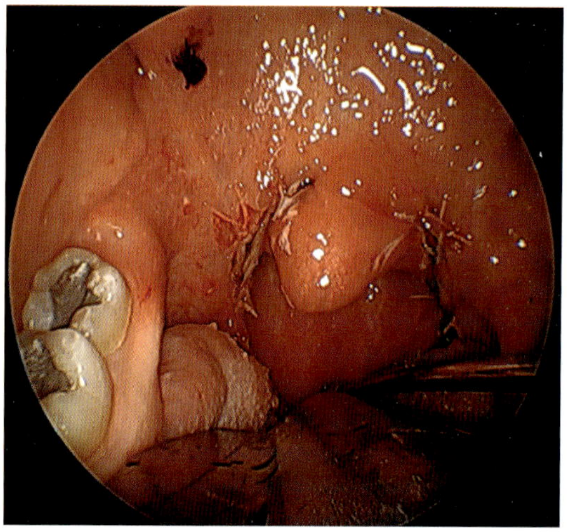

Fig. 9 Appearance of right tonsillar fossa after completion of one side of the pharyngoplasty procedure described above. Three 3-0 Vicryl sutures have been placed facilitating significant lateral pharyngeal wall expansion.

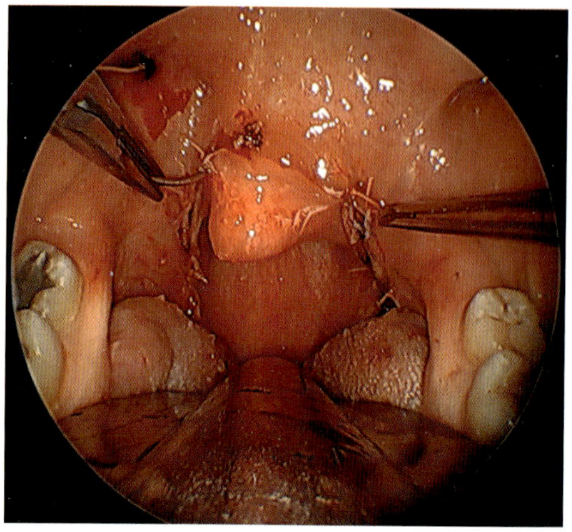

Fig. 11 The hamulus is carefully palpated with finger palpation and a horizontal mattress (vicryl needle on a CT-1 pop-off) is placed from lateral to medial in a 45-degree plane.

The appearance of bilateral pharyngeal walls after completion of tonsillectomy, uvulectomy, and bilateral pharyngoplasty is demonstrated in Figs. 10 and 11.

To complete the procedure and substantially improve anteroposterior expansion in the territory of the retrouvular space and velum, one suture in the form of a 2-0 Vicryl is placed from the hamulus to the base of the uvula (Fig 12).

These are performed in a horizontal-mattressed fashion beginning from the hamulus, extending to the uvula, and traversing back toward the hamulus before being snugly tied down (Fig. 13).

One suture is placed on each side of the palate, and the wounds are then double-checked to ensure hemostasis with gentle physical kneading of the tonsillar bed to ensure no bleeding is induced. A Valsalva maneuver can also be performed with the mouth prop let down to ensure an artificial tamponade effect is not observed (Fig. 14).

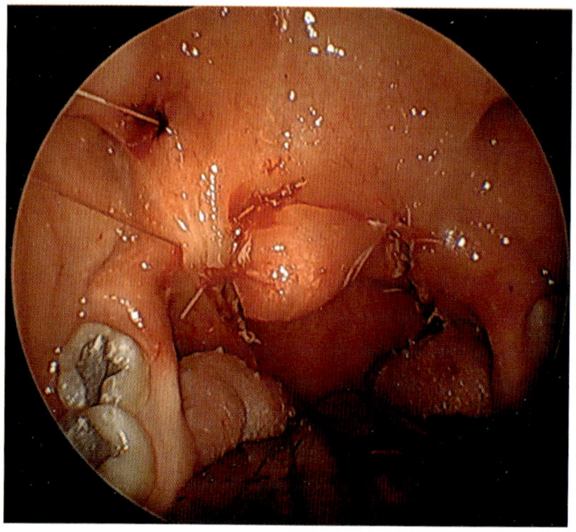

Fig. 12 The hamulus stitch allows suspension of the levator veli palatini.

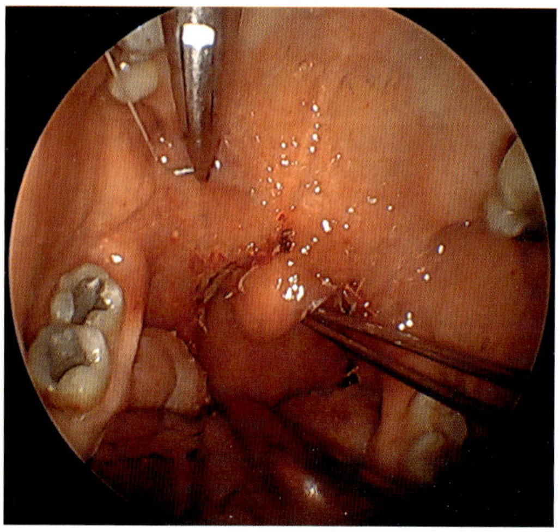

Fig. 10 Appearance of bilateral pharyngeal walls after completion of tonsillectomy, uvulectomy, and bilateral pharyngoplasty.

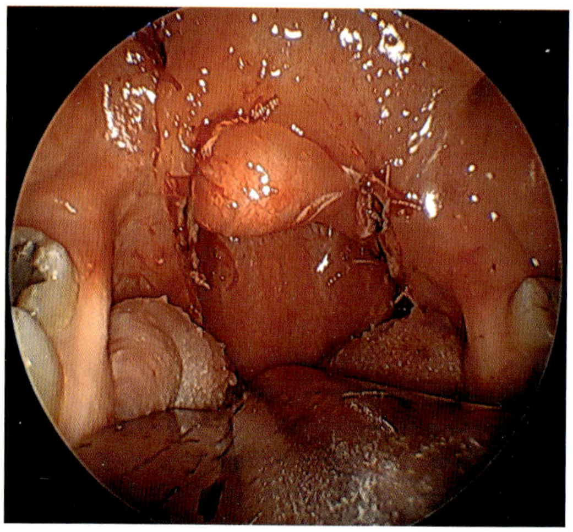

Fig. 13 This completes the procedure once repeated bilaterally and substantially improves anteroposterior expansion in the region of the retro-uvular space and velum.

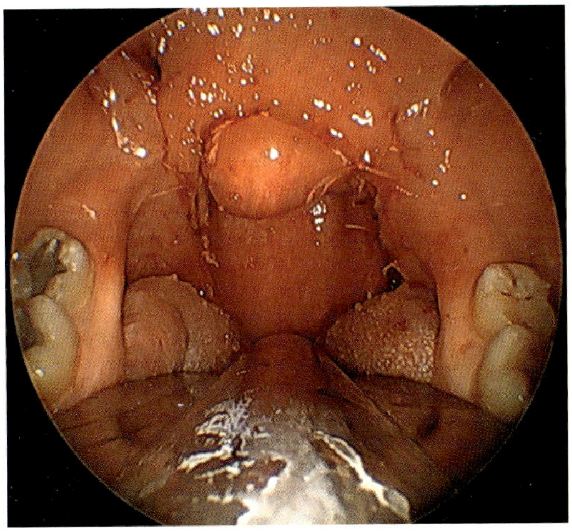

Fig. 14 Appearance of the palate and pharyngeal walls demonstrating substantial lateral pharyngeal wall, and antero-posterior expansion with reduction in uvular length and volume after completion of the procedure.

Potential complications

The complication rate following pharyngoplasty has routinely been demonstrated to be low.[10–13] Possible complications include swallowing disturbance, nasal regurgitation, voice change, persistent throat pain, airway embarrassment, and postoperative bleeding necessitating intervention. Major complications include laryngospasm, pulmonary edema, and postoperative desaturation. Minor complications include bleeding, uncontrolled pain, and nasopharyngeal insufficiency. Although perioperative mortalities have been reported, recent studies demonstrate no incidence of perioperative mortality following pharyngoplasty procedures, likely due to increased awareness of risk factors and reduced perioperative narcotic use.[14]

Postoperative care/rehabilitation and recovery

Numerous studies have argued that in appropriately selected patients, UPPP can be performed as outpatient surgery. At the authors' institution, patients are monitored for 24 hours postoperatively in a step-down unit before discharge. Oral antibiotics are administered for 7 days postoperatively and antinausea medications such as Dimenhydrinate or Ondansetron are prescribed to reduce postoperative nausea and emesis. In addition, stool softeners such as Lactulose and Senna are prescribed to reduce straining and associated risk of postoperative bleeding.

Clinical results

The value of UPPP has been previously questioned in the sleep medicine literature, beginning with Sher and colleagues' OSA surgery review, which demonstrated a success rate of 41% in all-comers. However, subset analysis demonstrated failure to identify the specific site of obstruction as the principal factor of poor surgical outcomes in this patient population. Of note, UPPP does provide benefit in outcomes such as motor vehicle accidents, cardiovascular disease, and overall mortality. Interestingly, UPPP has also been shown to provide improvements in sleep-related quality of life (Table 1).[15]

Table 1 Uvulopalatopharyngoplasty has been shown to provide improvements in sleep-related quality of life

Type I	Oropharyngeal narrowing with normal palatal arch
Type II	Low palatal arch and large tongue
Type IIa	Predominantly oropharynx with normal hypopharynx
Type IIb	Predominantly oropharynx with narrow hypopharynx
Type III	Normal oropharynx with compromised hypopharynx with large or posterior tongue, lateral wall bulge, hypertrophic lingual tonsils, and atonic supraglottis

Summary

Palatopharyngoplasty remains the most commonly performed surgical procedure for OSA worldwide.[16] Fifteen-year follow-up has shown significant and sustained reductions in oxygen desaturation index values ($ODI_{4\%}$). Two-thirds of patients fulfill criteria for surgical success ($ODI_{4\%}$ reduction of 50%, Apnea Hypopnea Index <20). No increase in mortality has been seen with most patients reporting improvement in excessive daytime sleepiness.[17] The procedure requires diligent preoperative patient selection for optimal success and remains of value in the sleep surgeon's armamentarium of soft tissue techniques.

Acknowledgments

The authors are indebted to Howard Awad, MD, ABSM for his assistance in reviewing and providing feedback on this article.

References

1. Schwab RJ, Gupta KB, Gefter WB, et al. Upper airway and soft tissue anatomy in normal subjects and patients with sleep-disordered breathing. Significance of the lateral pharyngeal walls. Am J Respir Crit Care Med 1995;152(5 Pt 1):1673–89.
2. Heinberg CJ. A surgical procedure for the relief of snoring. Eye Ear Nose Throat Mon 1955;34(6):389, passim.
3. Simmons FB, Guilleminault C, Silvestri R. Snoring, and some obstructive sleep apnea, can be cured by oropharyngeal surgery. Arch Otolaryngol 1983;109(8):503–7.
4. Fujita S, Conway W, Zorick F, et al. Surgical correction of anatomic abnormalities in obstructive sleep apnea syndrome: uvulopalatopharyngoplasty. Otolaryngol Head Neck Surg 2016; 89(6):923–34.
5. Certal V, Nishino N, Camacho M, et al. Reviewing the systematic reviews in OSA surgery. Otolaryngol Head Neck Surg 2013;149(6): 817–29.
6. Powell N, Riley R, Guilleminault C, et al. A reversible uvulopalatal flap for snoring and sleep apnea syndrome. Sleep 1996;19(7): 593–9.
7. Schellenberg JB, Maislin G, Schwab RJ. Physical findings and the risk for obstructive sleep apnea. The importance of oropharyngeal structures. Am J Respir Crit Care Med 2000;162(2 Pt 1): 740–8.
8. Cahali MB. Lateral pharyngoplasty: a new treatment for obstructive sleep apnea hypopnea syndrome. Laryngoscope 2003;113(11): 1961–8.

9. Pang KP, Woodson BT. Expansion sphincter pharyngoplasty: a new technique for the treatment of obstructive sleep apnea. Otolaryngol Head Neck Surg 2007;137(1):110–4.
10. Mickelson SA, Hakim I. Is postoperative intensive care monitoring necessary after uvulopalatopharyngoplasty? Otolaryngol Head Neck Surg 1998;119(4):352–6.
11. Spiegel JH, Raval TH. Overnight hospital stay is not always necessary after uvulopalatopharyngoplasty. Laryngoscope 2005; 115(1):167–71.
12. Kandasamy T, Wright ED, Fuller J, et al. The incidence of early postoperative complications following uvulopalatopharyngoplasty: identification of predictive risk factors. J Otolaryngol Head Neck Surg 2013;42(1):15.
13. Hathaway B, Johnson JT. Safety of uvulopalatopharyngoplasty as outpatient surgery. Otolaryngol Head Neck Surg 2006;134(4):542–4.
14. Pang KP. Identifying patients who need close monitoring during and after upper airway surgery for obstructive sleep apnoea. J Laryngol Otol 2006;120(8):655–60.
15. Weaver EM, Woodson BT, Yueh B, et al. Studying life effects & effectiveness of palatopharyngoplasty (SLEEP) study. Otolaryngol Head Neck Surg 2011;144(4):623–31.
16. Ishman SL, Ishii LE, Gourin CG. Temporal trends in sleep apnea surgery: 1993-2010. Laryngoscope 2014;124(5):1251–8.
17. Browaldh N, Friberg D, Svanborg E, et al. 15-year efficacy of uvulopalatopharyngoplasty based on objective and subjective data. Acta Otolaryngol 2011;131(12):1303–10.

Genioglossus and Genioplasty Advancement

Allen Cheng, DDS, MD, FACS [a,b,c,*]

KEYWORDS

- Genioplasty • Genioglossus advancement • Obstructive sleep apnea

KEY POINTS

- Genioglossus advancement with or without genioplasty is technique used as part of multilevel treatment of obstructive sleep apnea.
- Many modifications have been described to tailor the technique to patient and surgeon specifications.
- Computer-aided surgical planning and 3-dimensional printed guides remove much of the challenges of the surgery and allow for patient-specific osteotomy designs.

Introduction

Obstructive sleep apnea (OSA) is a complicated disease that is multifactorial. In many patients, obstruction at the level of the hypopharynx plays a prominent role. Examination of genioglossus activity in sleeping patients has identified progressive relaxation of tone culminating in obstructive events.[1] This suggests that the genioglossus muscle plays an important role in OSA.

Genioglossus advancement (GA), sometimes combined with hyoid suspension, is a surgery aimed at treating hypopharyngeal obstruction. It is often performed along with tonsillectomy, adenoidectomy, and uvulopalatopharyngoplasty as part of multilevel surgery. Because it is rarely performed in isolation, it is difficult to say how effective GA is in relieving hypopharyngeal obstruction and treating OSA. As part of multilevel surgery, analyses of case series (not controlled) have found success rates (defined as at least a 50% reduction in the Apnea-Hypopnea Index (AHI) and an AHI below 20) ranged between 40% and 70%.[2–5] A recent prospective study of patients with mild to moderate OSA receiving GA only has found similar success rates of 53%.[6]

Riley and colleagues[7] initially described GA as the inferior sagittal mandibular osteotomy. The ultimate goal was to advance the portion of the mandible that includes the genial tubercles, the attachment of the genioglossus muscle. Advancement of the genial tubercles is believed to tighten the genioglossus muscle, thereby mitigating relaxation and posterior positioning of the base of tongue and obstruction of the hypopharynx (Figs. 1 and 2). Since that time, there have been several modifications to this technique.

Modifications have included the anterior mandibular osteotomy, trephine osteotomy, genioplasty with genioglossus suspension suture, and combining anterior mandibular osteotomy with a genioplasty, among others.[8] Recent advances in computer-simulated surgery and 3-dimensional (3-D) printing of medical-grade cutting guides have allowed for patient-specific precision surgery on the inferior mandible.[9]

In this article, we review workup of patients for this procedure, indications and proper case selection, and a technique for performing GA with and without genioplasty. Complications also are discussed, to aid the reader in preoperative patient counseling.

Preoperative planning

The workup of a patient with OSA is discussed elsewhere in detail.[10] To briefly summarize, it starts with a careful history before moving onto physical examination. The focused examination of the head and neck should include a facial analysis, paying particular attention to the anterior-posterior and vertical development of the maxillomandibular complex.

A fiberoptic nasopharyngolaryngoscopy examination is a requisite part of the examination to identify the degree and level (or levels) of obstruction. Although helpful, awake upright fiberoptic examination does not accurately represent the conditions that occur with sleep-related obstructions.

If a patient is suspected of having a sleep disorder, a polysomnogram is performed to further characterize, diagnose, and grade the severity of the disorder.

Finally, a drug-induced sleep endoscopy is often a very helpful study that mitigates the limitations of an awake fiberoptic examination.

Indications

GA, alone or as part of a genioplasty, is typically one component of multilevel surgery to address OSA. The primary

Disclosure Statement: The author has nothing to disclose.

[a] Head and Neck Surgical Associates, 1849 Northwest Kearney Street, Suite 300, Portland, OR 97209, USA
[b] Oral/Head and Neck Oncology, Legacy Good Samaritan Cancer Center, 1015 North West, 22nd Avenue, Portland, OR 97210, USA
[c] Department of Oral and Maxillofacial Surgery, Oregon Health Sciences University, 2730 South West Moody Avenue, Portland, OR 97201, USA
* 1849 Northwest Kearney Street, Suite 300, Portland, OR 97209.
E-mail address: chenga@hnsa1.com

Atlas Oral Maxillofacial Surg Clin N Am 27 (2019) 23-28
1061-3315/19/
https://doi.org/10.1016/j.cxom.2018.11.008

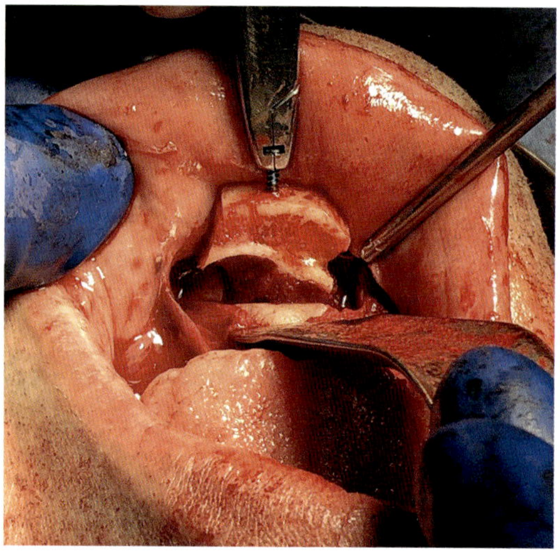

Fig. 1 Genioglossus muscle. (*Courtesy of* Stanley Y.C. Liu, MD, DDS, Stanford, CA.)

indication for GA is obstruction at the hypopharyngeal level, especially when associated with a retruded position of the base of tongue. Patients with mandibular retrognathism and retrogenia, in particular, benefit from GA with genioplasty, as it addresses both the hypopharyngeal obstruction and the dentofacial deformity.

Certain patients may have hypopharyngeal obstruction without significant or obvious retrognathism and retrogenia. These patients may not want the morphologic changes associated with an advancement genioplasty. In these circumstances, the anterior mandibular osteotomy should be considered.

As mentioned previously, there are limited data about the effectiveness of GA performed in isolation for treating OSA. The small number of studies examining the efficacy of GA have suggested that the technique, when performed without maxillomandibular advancement, was more likely to be effective in patients with mild to moderate OSA. As such, it is prudent to reserve isolated GA to patients with an AHI of 5 to 30.

Computer surgical planning

Traditionally, one of the more challenging parts of GA with genioplasty is performing the osteotomies in such a way that captures the genial tubercle and attachments of the genioglossus muscle. These osteotomies are performed from the labial cortex without being able to visualize the attachments that are on the lingual cortex. In addition, the apices of the mandibular incisors are in close proximity, making them at risk of injury by an errant saw blade. Several techniques have been described to allow for reliable approximation of the positioning of the osteotomies.[11] However, the advent of computer-aided surgical planning and 3-D printed tooth borne cutting guides has eliminated most of this risk. Because I use computer planning exclusively when planning this procedure, I will restrict my technique description to this approach.

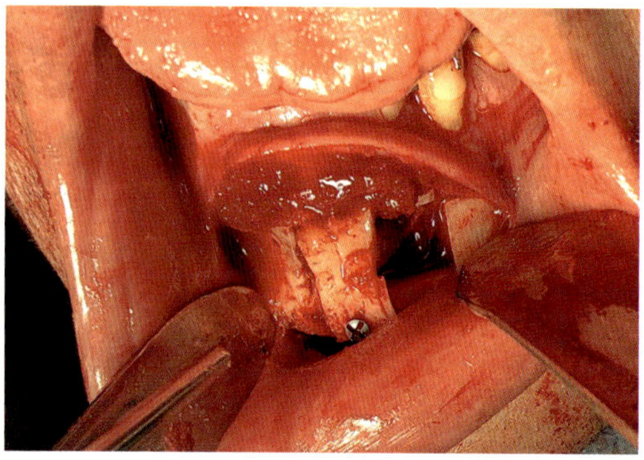

Fig. 2 Fixation with genioglossus muscle. (*Courtesy of* Stanley Y.C. Liu, MD, DDS, Stanford, CA.)

The digital work flow follows the clinical examination and includes a maxillofacial computed tomogram (CT) (Fig. 3). Although a medical-grade spiral CT with fine cuts is the most accurate, a cone-beam CT (CBCT) is serviceable, faster (when available), and exposes the patient to much less radiation. A dental impression is also taken. If an analog impression is used, this is poured up into a model. The model is scanned. Both the CBCT of the patient and dental models are sent electronically to the computer surgical planning company of choice. Previously, fiduciary occlusal wafers or jigs were required so that the model and facial CBCTs could be registered to each other, but current software algorithms allow for this to be performed accurately without this additional step. If digital impressions are taken, the file can be sent electronically.

Once received, the computer surgical planning is started with creation of 3D models and registration of the dental model to the maxillofacial model. Because CT imaging of the dentition is usually of poor resolution and obscured by restorative artifacts, the dental model is essential so that any tooth born guide will be accurate. This is performed off-line by the computer engineer.

A Web-based meeting is initiated. During this session, the surgeon and computer engineer plan the osteotomies and desired movements of the genioplasty segment. The ability to manipulate and visualize the lingual aspect of the mandible and the roots of the mandibular incisors is of tremendous utility. Because of this improved visualization, patient-specific osteotomies can be planned with a high degree of both accuracy and safety.[9]

There are some important considerations during the planning that should be observed. The first is identification of the genial tubercles. The second is highlighting the position of the mandibular incisors and canines. When planning for an anterior mandibular osteotomy (GA without genioplasty), the osteotomies must be parallel or diverging from lingual to labial, to allow the bone segment freedom to be drawn anteriorly. Finally, more or less of chin is included, depending on what would be more harmonious with the patient's facial form.

Once the Web meeting is completed, the remaining work is performed by the computer engineer off-line. A tooth borne cutting guide is designed, with guide planes for the saw cuts and predictive holes in the genioplasty segment (Fig. 4). For GA with genioplasty, a second positioning guide is designed with the desired advancement (Fig. 5). This is intended to be fixated to the genioplasty segment using the previously placed predictive holes. This allows for accurate replication of the desired planned movement.

Surgical approach

This procedure is typically performed either at a surgery center or operating room under general anesthesia, although also can

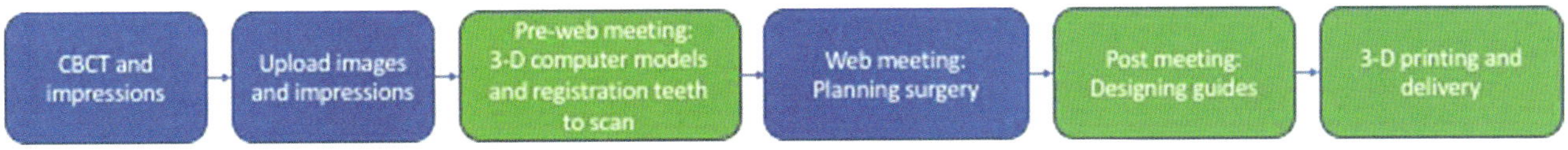

Fig. 3 Digital workflow for genioplasty. Blue boxes indicate steps performed by the surgeon. Green boxes indicate steps performed by computer engineers.

be performed under deep sedation, depending on surgeon and patient preference. Local anesthesia is used for bilateral mental nerve and lingual nerve blocks, along with generous infiltration.

I use a 15 blade to make a vestibular incision, 1.5 to 2.0 cm anterior to the mucogingival junction, through the labial mucosa. My nondominant hand holds the lower lip between thumb and index finger to provide tension. The index finger, placed on the skin, gives the surgeon a sense of the lip's thickness so as to avoid taking the dissection through the skin.

Using the blade (or electrocautery), I cut until the 2 bellies of the mentalis muscle are identified. The dissection is taken partially through the mentalis muscle, then redirected obliquely toward the mandibular bone. Doing so leaves a cuff of mentalis muscle on the other side of the incision. The dissection is then carried down to bone along a plane that is perpendicular to the alveolus of the mandible.

Once down to bone, a periosteal elevator is used to skeletonize the labial surface of the anterior mandible in a subperiosteal plane, down to the inferior border. This dissection is carried bilaterally along the inferior border until the mental nerve is identified on either side. This surgical approach has been described and illustrated extensively in other textbooks.[12]

Surgical procedure

Genioglossus advancement/anterior mandibular osteotomy

For a GA without genioplasty, also known as anterior mandibular osteotomy, the 3-D printed cutting guide is placed over the occlusal table of the mandibular teeth. It is essential to make sure that the occlusal portion of the guide is fully seated along the teeth and the bone guide is flush against the labial cortex of the anterior mandible. Using the appropriate drill for the desired fixation system, drill the predictive holes. Some systems use a drill guide to increase accuracy of the predictive holes. Fixation screws may be used to secure the guide to bone for further immobilization.

Once the guide is secured, a bicortical screw is placed through the advancement segment. A sagittal saw is then used to make the bicortical cuts through the mandible as marked by the guide planes. Typically, the segment is planned as a rectangular or trapezoidal shape. A spatula osteotome is used to complete the osteotomies. The segment is then drawn forward using a clamp placed on the bicortical screw. It is important that the screw used for traction engages both cortices so as to not separate the labial cortex from the lingual cortex.

Once the freed segment is pulled anteriorly, along with the genioglossus muscle, the fixation screw is removed. The labial cortex is then removed from the lingual cortex, which bears the attachment to the genioglossus. The lingual cortex is pulled anteriorly and fixated to the inferior border of the mandible using fixation plates and screws. Custom plates are very helpful for this, although add considerably to the material costs. The labial cortex that was previously removed may be secured to the osteotomy window to repair the defect. Alternatively, the rectangular lingual cortex can be rotated 90° in a coronal plane. The segment is secured to the bone superior and inferior to the bone window with fixation screws (Fig. 6).

Several modifications have been described for this technique. Rather than summarize the many multiple iterations of this technique, I highlight some notable modifications.

When computer planning and surgical guides are unavailable, the surgeon must rely on measurements based on anatomic landmarks. The genial tubercles are located 5 to 8 mm below the apices of the mandibular anterior teeth. This

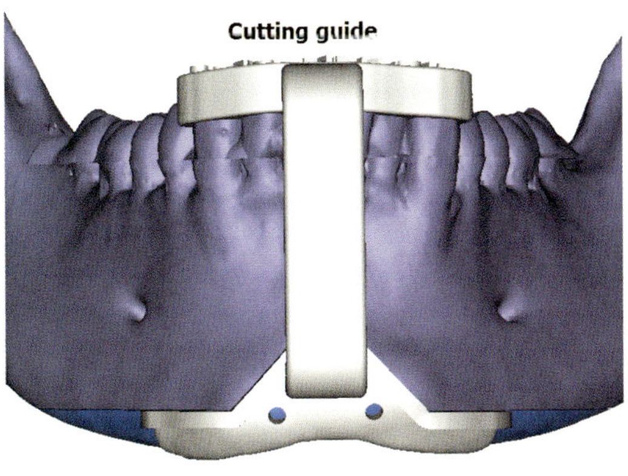

Fig. 4 Report showing computer planning and 3-D printed guides. Notice that the surgical guide has a plane meant to guide the location and angle of the reciprocating saw blade. Also, there are predictive holes meant for securing the second, positioning guide. (*Courtesy of* Rishi Jay Gupta, DDS, MD, MBA, San Francisco, CA.)

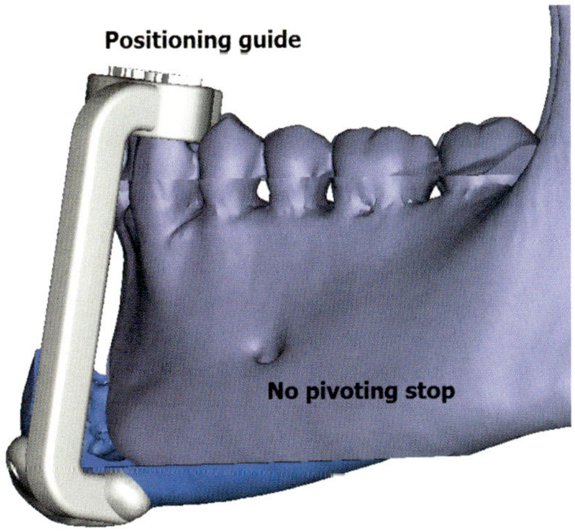

Fig. 5 Report showing the positioning guide, which is used to stabilize the genioplasty segment to allow for accurate fixation. (*Courtesy of* Rishi Jay Gupta, DDS, MD, MBA, San Francisco, CA.)

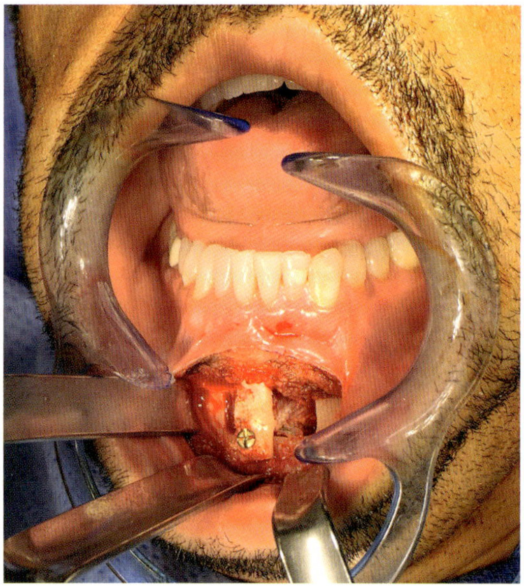

Fig. 6 Genioglossus segment advanced, labial cortex removed. The segment is then rotated 90° and secured to the native mandible. (*Courtesy of* Rishi Jay Gupta, DDS, MD, MBA, San Francisco, CA.)

can be easily confirmed by reviewing the patient's CT before surgery. The distance from the mandibular incisor roots and incisal edge to the genial tubercle is measured. The osteotomy is then planned to include the tubercle with a margin of safety from the root tips (Fig. 7).

An alternative method for GA is to first perform a traditional genioplasty osteotomy. With the genioplasty segment mobilized and retracted inferiorly, the genial tubercle and genioglossus attachments can be palpated and visualized. Once the genial tubercle is identified, either as part of the genioplasty segment or superiorly, a triangular or rectangular osteotomy can be performed to include it. This is pulled anteriorly and fixated to the mandible. The genioplasty segment is then fixated in the desired position with or without advancement.[13]

Genioglossus advancement with genioplasty

For GA with a genioplasty, also known as inferior sagittal mandibular osteotomy, the 3-D printed cutting guide is secured

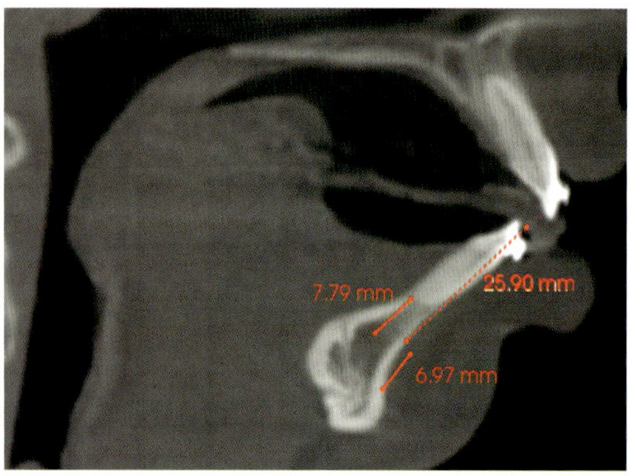

Fig. 7 Sagittal cut through the mandible. The distance is measured between the genial tubercle, the mandibular incisal edge, and the mandibular incisor root apices.

to the occlusal table, as described previously. Predictive holes are then drilled and positional screws are used to secure the guide to the bone. Two Langenback toe out retractors are used on either side to provide protection to the mental nerves. A sagittal saw is then used to make the horizontal osteotomy. This is most easily done cutting toward the midline from the opposite side. While making the osteotomies, it is essential to have a good sense of the depth of the blade, with the goal of making the cut in one pass, bicortical, but not so deep as to injure the genioglossus muscle bellies or the lingual vasculature. Because the osteotomies were planned using computer guidance, the surgeon can be confident that the tubercle is included in the genioplasty segment.

Once the osteotomy is completed, the guide is removed. An osteotome may be necessary to complete the osteotomy. Once freed, the second, positioning guide is secured to the teeth and fixated to the genioplasty segment, using the same holes made previously. The guide is designed with the planned advancement, as well as to leave space for placement of a fixation plate.

I usually use a pre-bent genioplasty plate. It is simple and efficient to use, and has greater strength than a plate that is bent to the same shape. Alternatively, many of the craniomaxillofacial hardware companies are now able to fashion custom hardware (Fig. 8). This makes the positioning and fixation of the genioplasty segment significantly easier by removing the need for the second positioning guide. All that is necessary is accurate predictive holes on both the proximal mandible and genioplasty segment. In addition, the strength and rigidity of custom plates are similar to reconstruction plates.

Closure

The wound is thoroughly irrigated with normal saline to wash out debris. I take the time to inspect the surgical site for hemostasis, particularly in the area of the osteotomies. Inadvertent injury to the sublingual artery and veins by a reciprocating saw can easily occur. It is important to identify this and address this at the time of surgery to avoid sublingual hematoma formation.

The closure starts with suspension of the 2 bellies of the mentalis muscle. This is done with three 4-0 Vicryl (or equivalent) sutures. It is helpful to pass all 3 sutures before tying them down to facilitate accurate approximation of the muscle bellies. Accurate muscle closure is essential to avoid chin ptosis and gingival recession around the mandibular teeth.

A running 3-0 chromic gut suture is used to close the mucosa in a second layer. I prefer a horizontal mattress for improved eversion of the mucosa edges. I do not leave drains in the wound.

An Elastoplast (or Tensoplast) dressing is placed, with adhesive, externally on the skin over the chin. This provides external compression to aid in hemostasis and prevent hematoma formation. This is removed on the second postoperative day.

Potential complications

GA with or without genioplasty is a low-risk surgery; however, there are a number of potential complications to review with the patient during the consultation period.

Neurosensory dysfunction is the most common complication, although usually this is transient. Given the minimal

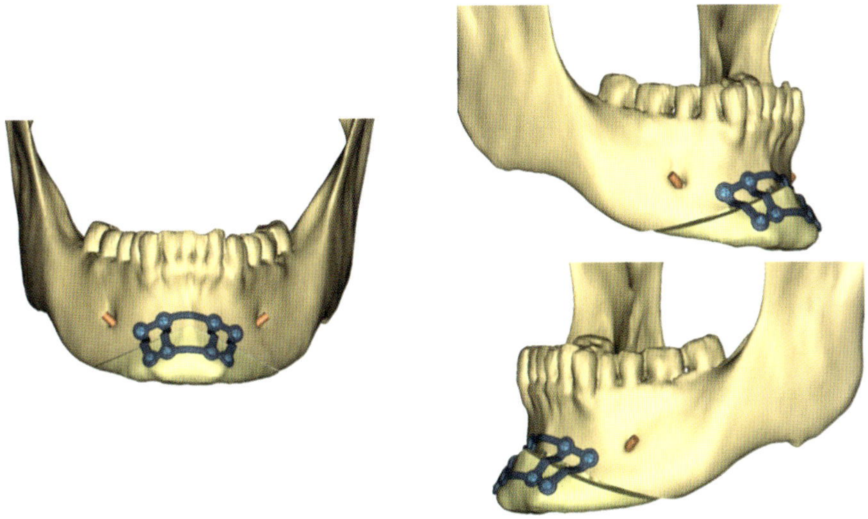

Fig. 8 Example of a custom genioplasty advancement plate. (*Courtesy of* Rishi Jay Gupta, DDS, MD, MBA, San Francisco, CA.)

dissection around the mental nerve, long-term neurosensory dysfunction is unlikely. The patient should be prepared for this. In addition, many patients report altered sensation of the mandibular incisor teeth.

Local infection is not uncommon and is managed with minimally invasive measures. I do use and recommend preoperative antibiotics. The efficacy of postoperative antibiotics is debatable.[14] I prescribe these on a case-by-case basis. I do routinely prescribe postoperative chlorhexidine mouth rinse, although there is also a dearth of evidence for or against this.

Wound dehiscence is another common minor complication. This is managed conservatively with wound cleansing. I supply my patients with a Monojet syringe and instruct them to gently rinse the wound with salt water after meals. I have the patients continue chlorhexidine rinses until the wound closes. I do not make any attempts to close these wounds, as this is futile. Occasionally, wound dehiscence results in persistent hardware exposure. Exposed hardware is kept clean with oral hygiene and chlorhexidine rinses. Hardware is removed after bony union has been confirmed.

Gingival recession around the mandibular incisors can occur when the mentalis is not suspended during closure. The wound contracture that occurs with inadequate mentalis suspension causes downward tensile forces on the gingival soft tissue, resulting in recession. This is avoidable with meticulous closure.

Injury to the mandibular incisors and canines is also a rare, and generally avoidable, complication. This most easily occurs during using a saw to make the osteotomy. This is often of little consequence. On occasion, these teeth may require endodontic treatment. If root injury is suspected, these teeth are monitored clinically and radiographically, as manifestation of necrotic teeth may take some time before they can be diagnosed. Furthermore, interpretation of vitality testing is complicated by neurosensory dysfunction, which may take considerable time to recuperate.

Dehiscence of the genioglossus muscle from the mandible is a rare complication due to excessive force applied to the mobilized segment or unintentional dissection of the lingual soft tissue. This is difficult to diagnose, but would result in failure of the surgery to relieve the hypopharyngeal obstruction.

When the inferior mandibular sagittal osteotomy (genioplasty) was described as a technique in lieu of maxillomandibular advancement and became widely adopted, some surgeons reported instances of midline mandible fracture. Because of the loss of the horizontal buttress of the anterior mandible, masticatory forces were believed to fracture the weaker alveolar bone. Because of this, some surgeons have recommended a 6-week period of a soft mechanical diet to avoid excessive masticatory forces.[8] In addition, some surgeons have advocated reinforcing the mandible with a load-bearing reconstruction plate. However, this complication is exceedingly rare, made more so by the advent of precision surgery using computer planning. I restrict diet to a soft mechanical diet for the first 2 weeks.

Pearls and pitfalls

- Facial analysis, in particular studying the relationship of the mandible to the maxilla, the chin point to the lower incisor position, and the facial profile, is essential for deciding between GA with or without genioplasty.
- During the surgical approach, be sure to include a cuff of mentalis on the mandibular side of the incision to aid in resuspension of that muscle. This will help avoid chin ptosis and gingival recession.
- Computer planning can expedite the surgery and allow for precision osteotomies that avoid injury to tooth roots while ensuring capture of the genial tubercles.
- When computer planning is not available, careful analysis of the sagittal sections of a facial CT will help with planning the osteotomies.

Immediate postoperative care

GA and genioplasty, when performed in isolation, are generally outpatient procedures. However, given the nature of the disease and location of the surgery, there is concern for floor of mouth and tongue swelling that may lead to airway embarrassment. To avoid this, careful postoperative instructions are given to the patient to watch out for signs and symptoms of sublingual hematoma. These would include dysphagia, odynophagia, sialorrhea (from inability to swallow secretions), dyspnea, a raised floor of mouth, and protruding tongue. The patient should return for follow-up in 1 to 2 weeks.

Oral hygiene is paramount. Patients should be specifically instructed to continue with normal dental hygiene, to rinse their mouths gently after meals, and to adhere to a soft diet. I do prescribe chlorhexidine 0.12% oral rinse to be used twice daily for the first week.

Patients should be counseled to expect some swelling and bruising. In older patients and those with fair skin, it is not unusual to have bruising that extends from the submental region down onto the chest. Preparing patients for this will save them from unnecessary duress.

Pain is managed according to the surgeon's preferences, but I generally recommend a combination of nonsteroidal anti-inflammatory drugs (ibuprofen) and acetaminophen. I do prescribe a small amount of opioid combination medications (hydrocodone/acetaminophen), although I counsel the patient to minimize use of these medications and reserve them only for extreme breakthrough pain.

Rehabilitation and recovery

Generally, these are very well tolerated procedures. The first 2 weeks, patients should be counseled to expect pain and swelling. I counsel patients to anticipate taking several days from work, more if the patient has a physically demanding occupation. I also prepare them that it typically takes 2 weeks for full recovery, to help them gauge the amount of their own specific post-operative convalescence that they think they may require.

Summary

GA with or without genioplasty is a surgery that is an important technique for the sleep surgeon's armamentarium. It is typically one component of multilevel surgery. The technique, particularly when performed in isolation, should be reserved for patients with mild to moderate OSA to maintain a reasonable chance of success. The advent of CT imaging, computer planning, 3-D printing, and custom hardware have all made it easier to avoid complications such as dental injury and dehiscence of the genioglossus muscle.

References

1. Adachi S, Lowe AA, Tsuchiya M, et al. Genioglossus muscle activity and inspiratory timing in obstructive sleep apnea. Am J Orthod Dentofacial Orthop 1993;104(2):138–45.
2. Riley RW, Powell NB, Guilleminault C. Obstructive sleep apnea syndrome: a review of 306 consecutively treated surgical patients. Otolaryngol Head Neck Surg 1993;108(2):117–25.
3. Vilaseca I, Morelló A, Montserrat JM, et al. Usefulness of uvulopalatopharyngoplasty with genioglossus and hyoid advancement in the treatment of obstructive sleep apnea. Arch Otolaryngol Head Neck Surg 2002;128(4):435–40.
4. Ramirez SG, Loube DI. Inferior sagittal osteotomy with hyoid bone suspension for obese patients with sleep apnea. Arch Otolaryngol Head Neck Surg 1996;122(9):953–7.
5. Lee NR, Givens CD, Wilson J, et al. Staged surgical treatment of obstructive sleep apnea syndrome: a review of 35 patients. J Oral Maxillofac Surg 1999;57(4):382–5.
6. KuŞÇu O, Süslü AE, Özer S, et al. Sole effect of genioglossus advancement on apnea hypopnea index of patients with obstructive sleep apnea. Acta Otolaryngol 2015;135(8):835–9.
7. Riley RW, Powell NB, Guilleminault C. Inferior sagittal osteotomy of the mandible with hyoid myotomy-suspension: a new procedure for obstructive sleep apnea. Otolaryngol Head Neck Surg 1986; 94(5):589–93.
8. Lee NR. Genioglossus muscle advancement techniques for obstructive sleep apnea. Oral Maxillofac Surg Clin North Am 2002; 14(3):377–84.
9. Liu SY-C, Huon L-K, Zaghi S, et al. An accurate method of designing and performing individual-specific genioglossus advancement. Otolaryngol Head Neck Surg 2017;156(1):194–7.
10. Lee NR. Evaluation of the obstructive sleep apnea patient and management of snoring. Oral Maxillofac Surg Clin North Am 2009; 21(4):377–87.
11. Lee NR, Madani M. Genioglossus muscle advancement techniques for obstructive sleep apnea. Atlas Oral Maxillofac Surg Clin North Am 2007;15(2):179–92.
12. Ellis E, Zide MF. Surgical approaches to the facial skeleton. Lippincott Williams & Wilkins; 2015.
13. Rojas R, Chateau R, Gaete C, et al. Genioglossus muscle advancement and simultaneous sliding genioplasty in the management of sleep apnoea. Int J Oral Maxillofac Surg 2018;47(5): 638–41.
14. Oomens MAEM, Verlinden CRA, Goey Y, et al. Prescribing antibiotic prophylaxis in orthognathic surgery: a systematic review. Int J Oral Maxillofac Surg 2014;43(6):725–31.

Maxillomandibular Advancement

Contemporary Approach at Stanford

Stanley Yung-Chuan Liu, MD, DDS [a,*], Michael Awad, MD, FRCSC [b], Robert Wayne Riley, MD, DDS [a]

KEYWORDS

• Obstructive sleep apnea • Maxillomandibular advancement • Facial skeletal surgery • Counterclockwise rotation • Lateral wall stabilization

KEY POINTS

- Maxillomandibular advancement (MMA) demonstrates consistently high surgical success and modest cure rates for patients with obstructive sleep apnea (OSA).
- Indications for MMA as first-line surgical treatment include patients with preexisting dentofacial deformity, severe OSA, and airway collapse pattern (complete centric at velum, and complete at lateral pharyngeal wall) examined by drug-induced sedation endoscopy (DISE).
- MMA involves a counterclockwise rotation with the center at the maxillary buttress to maximize airway muscle tension and balance facial esthetics.
- Technique modifications from routine orthognathic surgery for MMA are important to address both surgical and patient related factors.

Video content accompanies this article at http://www.oralmaxsurgeryatlas.theclinics.com.

Introduction: nature of the problem

Since the authors' first review of 40 patients undergoing maxillomandibular advancement (MMA), a procedure pioneered at Stanford Hospital for the treatment of obstructive sleep apnea (OSA), MMA has remained one of the most effective and reliable surgical intervention for OSA, with its high surgical success rate.[1–5]

In the early years, MMA was part of a 2-phase algorithm where phase 1 (palate, nasal, tongue base procedures, hyoid advancement, and genioglossus advancement) was followed by phase 2 (MMA) in cases of treatment resistance. The earliest indications for MMA included severe OSAS, morbid obesity, severe mandibular deficiency, and failure of other forms of therapy.[6,7]

Today, selection criteria for MMA includes the use of dynamic examination, such as drug-induced sleep endoscopy (DISE). MMA is particularly effective in treating OSA patients with lateral pharyngeal wall and concentric velum collapse during DISE. Severe OSA patients with this collapse pattern tend to have low hyoid position, as shown with sleep MRI.[8] Because concentric collapse of the velum is contraindicated in upper airway (hypoglossal) stimulation, and lateral pharyngeal wall collapse is difficult to address with soft tissue pharyngeal procedures,[9,10] MMA can be a first-line recommendation in OSA patients with this dynamic airway collapse pattern.

MMA is also performed in OSA patients with dentofacial deformity. However, in patients with Class 1 skeletal relationship, MMA with airway-specific counterclockwise (CCW) rotation can be expeditiously performed with minimal orthodontic decompensation.

The role of MMA in reducing the burden of disease in OSA is an important distinction from previous representations where surgical cure was the primary outcome. A favorable outcome is one that mitigates patient symptoms and comorbid risk, with improved quality of life reflected by high levels of patient satisfaction. MMA need not be the only intervention; the authors have performed soft tissue pharyngeal surgery and hypoglossal nerve stimulation to achieve overall treatment success (cure).

There are ample texts that describe the basics of jaw surgery which involve Le Fort I and sagittal split osteotomies. This Atlas article focuses on key steps that define the Stanford MMA. These steps are founded on 3 decades of experience with Nelson B. Powell and Robert W. Riley. Contemporary extension of their philosophy from breathing-focused to bite (brevity of orthodontic treatment with surgery-first protocol) and beauty (balance of facial proportions including nasal form and function) by Stanley Y.C. Liu is also highlighted.

Disclosure Statement: The authors have nothing to disclose.

[a] Division of Sleep Surgery, Department of Otolaryngology, Stanford Sleep Surgery Fellowship, Stanford University School of Medicine, 801 Welch Road, Stanford, CA 94304, USA

[b] Division of Sleep Surgery, Department of Otolaryngology—Head and Neck Surgery, Stanford University School of Medicine, Stanford Hospital and Clinics, 801 Welch Road, Stanford, CA 95304, USA

* Corresponding author.

E-mail address: ycliu@stanford.edu

Atlas Oral Maxillofacial Surg Clin N Am 27 (2019) 29-36

https://doi.org/10.1016/j.cxom.2018.11.011

Surgical technique

Preoperative planning

Appropriate patient selection begins with a thorough history, subjective questionnaires (Epworth Sleepiness Scale and Nasal Obstructive Symptom Evaluation), head and neck physical examination, polysomnography interpretation, and fiberoptic nasopharyngoscopy observation. Selectively DISE is used. These objective and subjective examinations can be used in combination with CT imaging to identify appropriate skeletal surgery patients and plan procedures.

The most unique aspect of today's Stanford MMA in preoperative planning is the center of rotation for the maxillomandibular complex (MMC). Although it is a CCW rotation, the center of rotation is uniquely placed to maximize both airway stability and facial esthetics. Additionally, the main reference points and movements for planning are (1) advancement from a point at the piriform rim just below level of the inferior turbinate, (2) degree of occlusal plane change dictated by the maxilla, and (3) postoperative position of the pogonion. If patients also exhibit dentofacial deformity, this is certainly addressed, but the general principle of movement, as described here remains consistent.

Prior to virtual surgical planning (VSP), Riley and Powell performed what is commonly described in the cosmetic maxillofacial literature as a single-splint technique.[11] This requires extensive experience to control the pitch, roll, and yaw of the MMC and is difficult to reproduce consistently by junior surgeons.

With VSP, surgical movements are planned, and 2 intermediate splints are usually produced to maximize the freedom to balance facial and airway position intraoperatively. Regarding the movement, a differential anterior impaction is performed with the rotation center in line with the buttress. CCW rotation has been described with centers at the anterior nasal spine (ANS) or posterior nasal spine (PNS). The buttress may seem like a peculiar landmark. The rationale is that when the maxilla is rotated in line with the buttress and the level of first molar is maintained, the CCW rotation actually brings the entire maxilla posterior to the original piriform rim. From here, an advancement of approximatley 3-mm to 5-mm anterior to the piriform translates to a final pogonion position approximately 12-mm to 18-mm anterior and 2-mm to 4-mm superior to its original position. The maxillary occlusal plane rotates in CCW direction by approximately 6° to 10°. Attention is given to correction of concurrent orthognathic problems if present (ie, mandibular asymmetry or class 2 or class 3 discrepancy). Notice that the surgery is not planned based on classic cephalometric measures, such as the SNA and SNB. The MMA movements, as described here advance and rotate the MMC to optimize airway and esthetic outcome.

In the representative VSP plan shown in Fig. 1, there is an occlusal plane change of 11° in a CCW fashion. This is planned via a 3-mm impaction at the piriform rim, while keeping the center of rotation at the buttress. The maxilla is then advanced just 5-mm anterior to the piriform rim. This movement results in a 12-mm advancement at the incisor, 7.6-mm advancement of the A point, 15.7-mm advancement of the B point, and a 23.5-mm advancement of the pogonion (Fig. 1).

This MMA patient in Fig. 2 underwent a similar movement. Due to the relatively small change at the midface coupled with piriformplasty and intraoperative septoplasty, his midfacial balance is not compromised. At the same time, note the significant advancement of the mandible, which is discernible both in the clinical photo and the immediate postoperative CT in the lateral view (Figs. 2 and 3).

Preparation and patient positioning

There are 2 important nuances to the positioning of the MMA patient compared with the orthognathic patient.

Classically, nasal RAE tubes are popular for orthognathic cases. OSA patients, however, tend to have longer airways. This requires a longer tube, but the longer RAE (Ring, Adair and Elwyn) tubes have larger diameter lumens. This significantly distorts the nasal anatomy such that intraoperative septoplasty and piriformplasty are difficult to perform with accuracy. Instead, the authors use the microlaryngoscopy tube (MLT), where there is adequate length, and thinner diameters, such as a 5.0 mm or 6.0 mm. The authors trim back the tube toward the nares and place a 120° reverse metallic attachment, followed in-line with an accordion extension.

Patients are not placed on a shoulder roll because this tends to further extend the neck. The authors leave patients in their

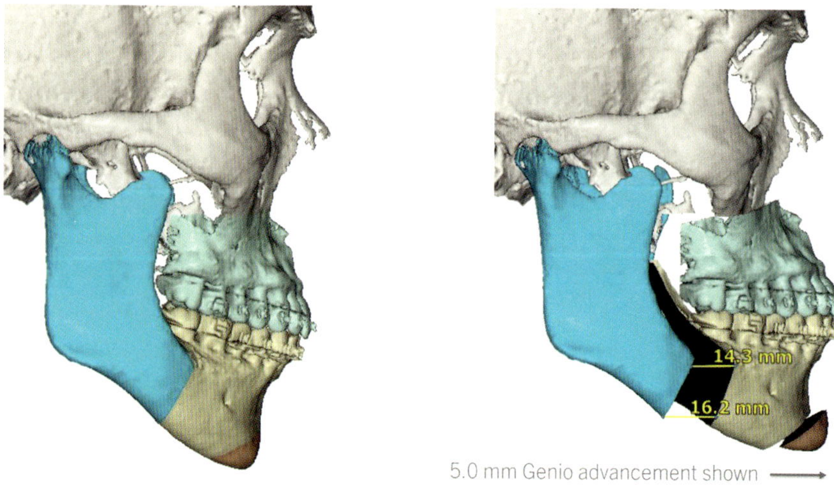

Fig. 1 VSP with CCW rotation centered at buttress (*left panel*, Before MMA; *right panel*, After MMA).

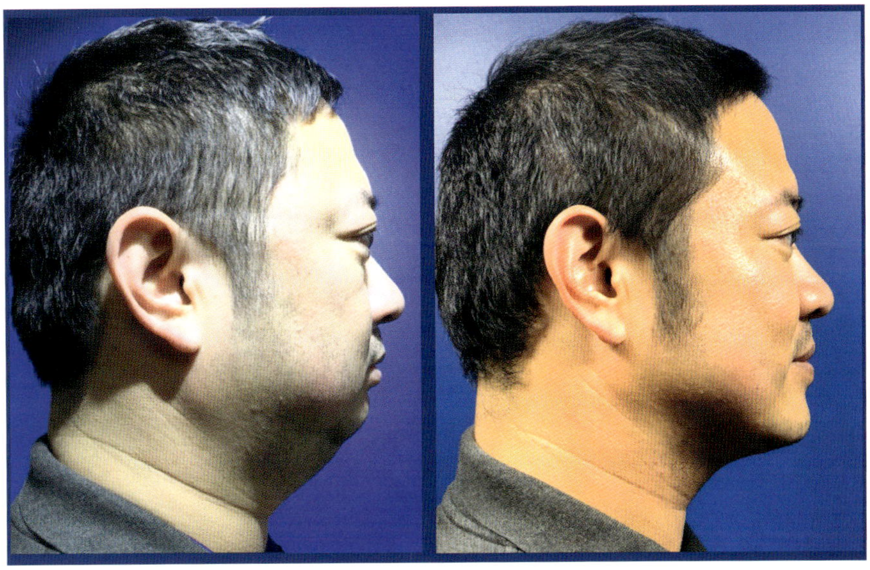

Fig. 2 MMA patient before (*left panel*) and after (*right panel*).

natural head position. This is important for control of the occlusal plane change (Fig. 4).

Anesthetic approach/sedation agent

Total intravenous anesthesia with agents such as propofol and remifentanil, is used. Although controlled hypotension with a target mean arterial pressure of 60 mm Hg is recommended for orthognathic procedures, in reality many MMA patients have significant cardiovascular comorbidities. Keeping the mean arterial pressure this low is both difficult for the anesthesiologist and contraindicated for some of the patients. The authors still aim for a brief period of controlled hypotension during maxillary down-fracture but most often are doing this at a mean arterial pressure of approximately 80 mm Hg. Total blood loss is approximately 250 mL to 350 mL for the procedure.

Although the authors' severe OSA patients are observed in the ICU for the first evening, all patients are extubated at the end of procedure. The authors work closely with anesthesia colleagues during extubation to help with nasal and oral suctioning. Postoperatively, the MMA patients are placed in light guiding elastics with no intraoral splint. This allows easy mouth opening in an emergent situation.

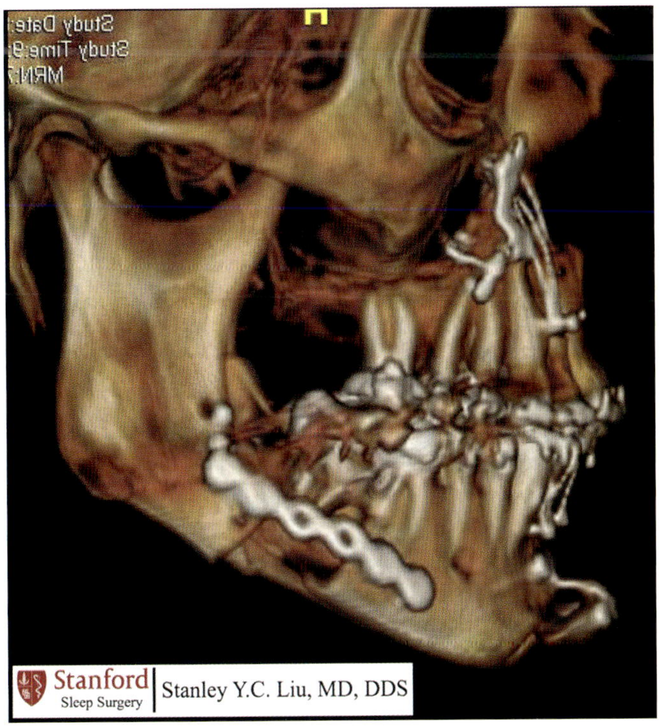

Fig. 3 Postoperative CT after MMA. Suspension wires are removed 6 weeks after surgery.

Surgical procedure

Approach to general aspects of MMA surgery is not discussed in detail. Instead, critical key steps are highlighted.

At the time of Le Fort I osteotomy, a wedge is created that determines the degree of CCW rotation. An appropriate degree of CCW rotation should not compromise incisor show in the final maxillary position.

The maxilla is never mobilized aggressively with instruments like the Rowe disimpaction forceps (Sklar Surgical Instruments, West Chester, PA). With a wire through the anterior nasal spine area to control the maxilla, lateral forces are applied concurrently to the posterior maxillary wall to mobilize the maxilla (Video 1). The usual anterior pull by the disimpaction forceps is especially ineffectively against previously operated soft

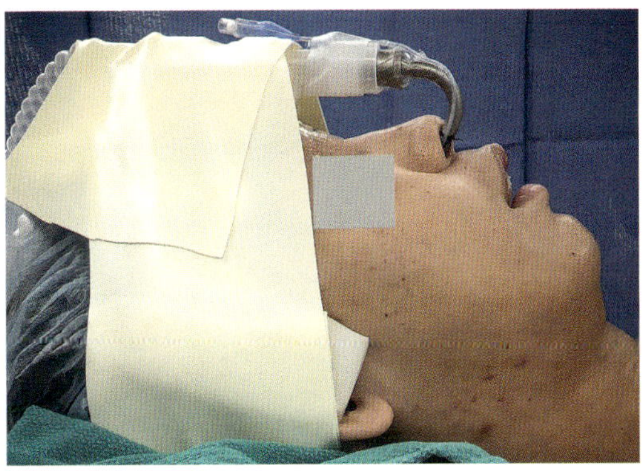

Fig. 4 Nasal intubation 120° metal connector.

palate. Large degree of torque by the disimpaction forceps is also uncontrolled, particularly in the average MMA patient, who tends to be an older adult.

With large CCW rotations, muscle tension associated with the maxilla and mandible is significant. For this reason, maxillomandibular fixation prior to rigid fixation is performed with the aid of suspension wires. The authors use suspension wires anchored to the alveolus with a 2.0-mm screw and through a hole by the piriform rim above the Le Fort osteotomy for the maxilla, and to the arch wire for the mandible. Maxillomandibular fixation prior to fixation with the use of 24-gauge wires on dental brackets or the arch bar would debond brackets or shift the arch bar. Minor discrepancy greatly affects accuracy of the final fixation.

The authors do not perform sagittal split osteotomy with instruments like Smith spreaders. Older patients tend to have little bone marrow space. With the need of longer osteotomy (anterior extent to the second premolar) for fixation after large advancements, the use of Smith spreaders lead to poorly controlled fractures. Instead, the authors focus on an accurate horizontal osteotomy just beyond the lingula, anterior osteotomy not past the inferior midline of mandible, and a wedging open of segments with 3 osteotomes in a sequential sandwiched fashion (Fig. 13).

Finally, with fixation, the authors use 2 to 3 bicortical fixation screws, coupled with a long 2.4-mm plate across the osteotomy site. The rigidity allows the patient a rapid return to function. Patients generally are not kept in a splint, and only light guiding elastics are used immediately after surgery. This allows MMA patients to breathe orally in the immediate post-operative period. By the end of the second week postoperatively, patients begin a pureed to soft diet. Minimal use of narcotic pain medications is expected.

Surgical steps

1. Le Fort osteotomy is followed by a wedge taken at the anterior piriform rim, with rotation center at the maxillary buttress (Figs. 5 and 6).

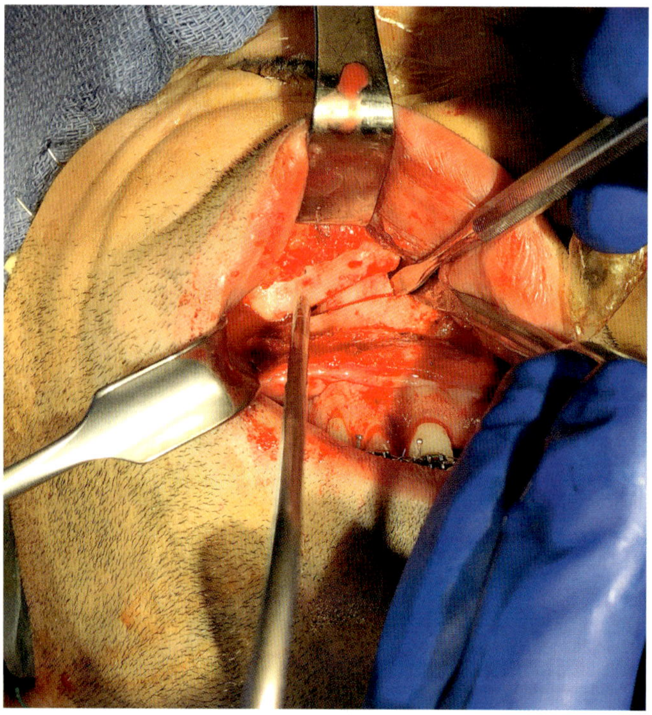

Fig. 5 Le Fort I wedge for counter clockwise rotation.

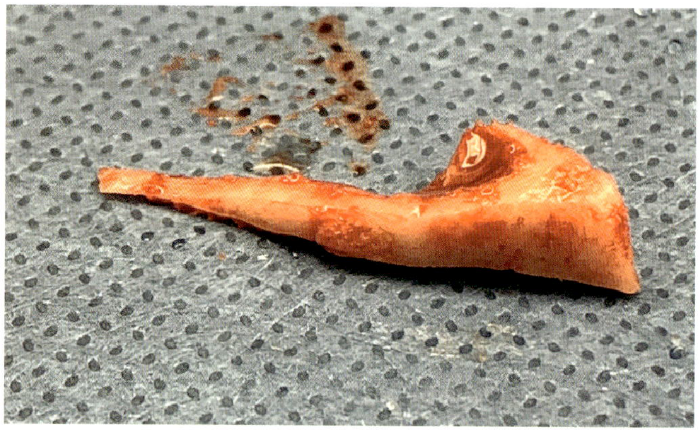

Fig. 6 Wedge removed.

2. A wire is passed through the anterior nasal spine to control the maxilla.
3. Specially designed gentle distractor is placed behind the posterior maxilla, anterior to the sphenoid bone (Video 1).
4. Descending palatine artery is identified and preserved (Fig. 7).
5. Maxillary mobility is ensured (Video 2).
6. Septoplasty is performed. The nasal floor is widened with a pineapple bur. The piriform rim is widened. The inferior turbinates are reduced with radiofrequency ablation, followed by outfracture. They are never resected entirely as classically described in orthognathic literature, to prevent atrophic rhinitis (Fig. 8, Video 3).
7. Frequently, OSA patients have chronic sinusitis with polyps. This is removed (Fig. 9).
8. Intermediate splint is placed, and measurements taken to ensure no cant has been introduced.
9. Preformed step-plates or custom plates are used to fixate the maxilla.
10. Suspension wires are placed, looping around a hole in the lateral piriform rim above the level of Le Fort I osteotomy, to a 11-mm or 13-mm screw placed in the alveolus. For the mandible, the wire wraps around the arch wire/ arch bar, to a similar alveolus screw. These wires later are used to perform maxillomandibular fixation prior to

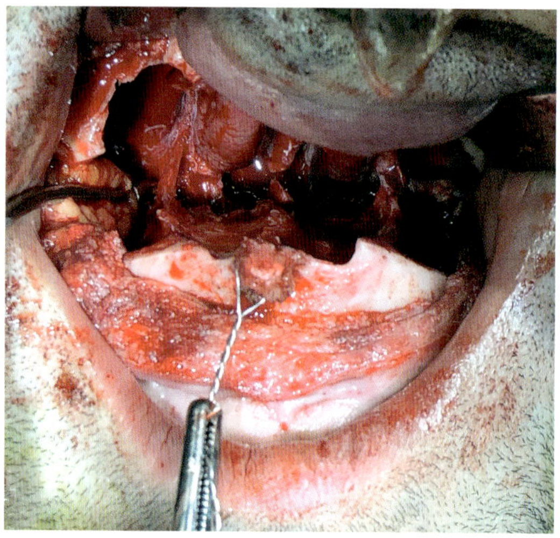

Fig. 7 Control of the maxilla via wire through anterior nasal spine. Descending palatine arteries are visualized bilaterally.

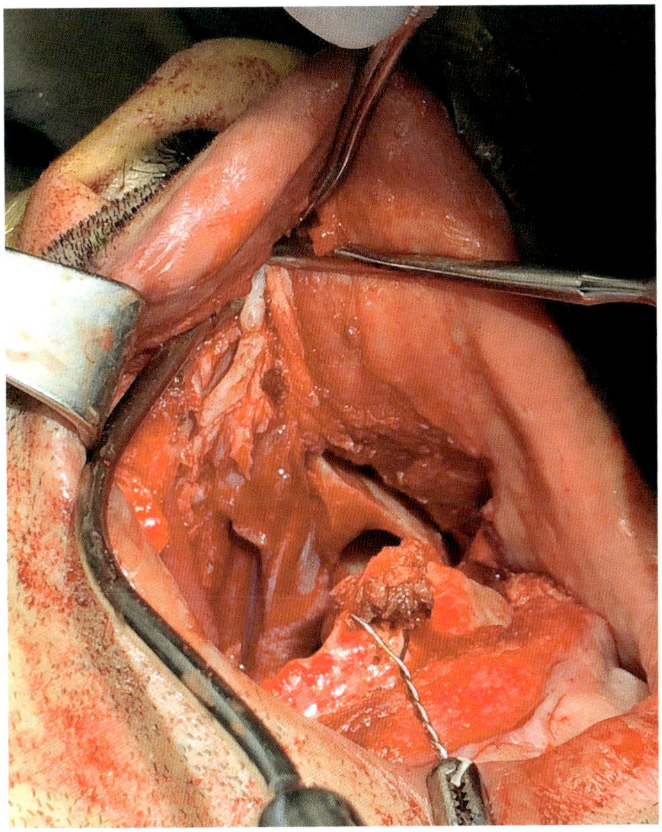

Fig. 8 Septum exposed.

application of mandibular bicortical screw and plates (Fig. 10).

11. Assessment of degree of maxillary advancement achieved (Video 4).

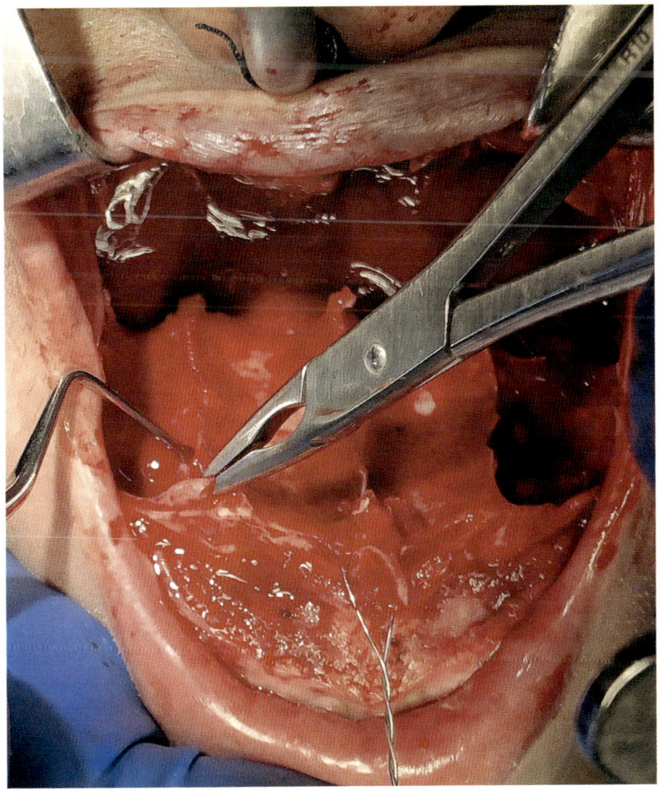

Fig. 9 Removal of maxillary sinus polyp.

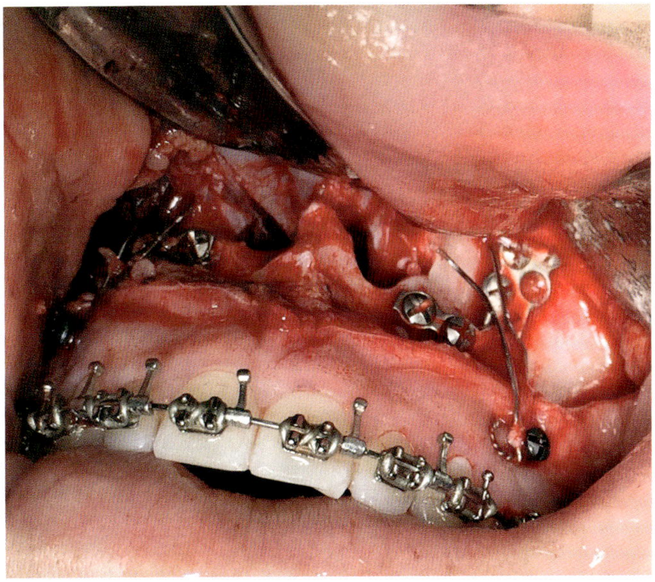

Fig. 10 Maxillary suspension wire.

12. If genioglossus advancement is planned, this precedes sagittal osteotomy. The authors prefer VSP-guided genial osteotomy that includes the inferior border of the anterior mandible, with superior extension to the genial tubercles. This ensures both capture of the genioglossus and suprahyoid muscles. Generous mentalis muscle cuff is important for coverage of the advancement plates and significant advancement of the bone graft (generally 7–9 mm) (Fig. 11).
13. Medial wall toward the lingula is burred down with a pineapple bur. This ensures a clear path to the lingula and

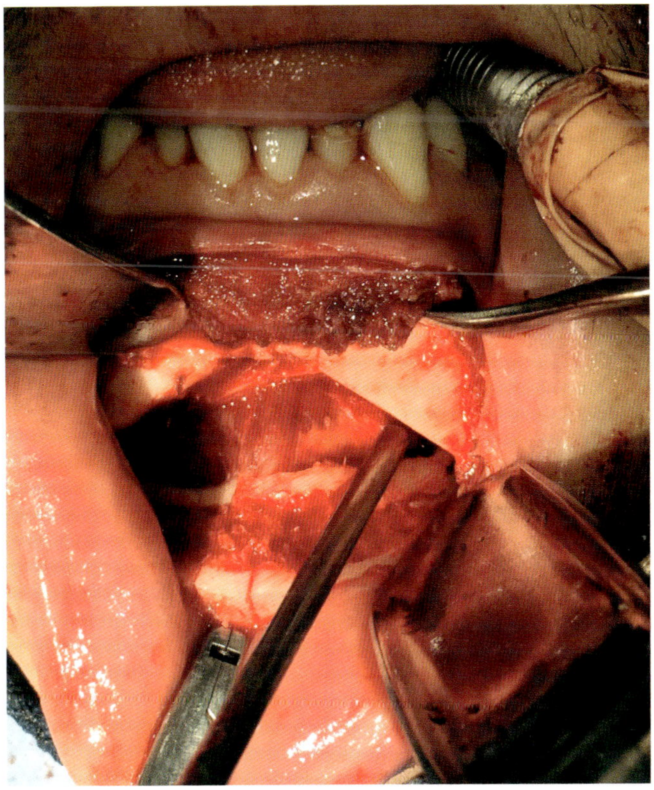

Fig. 11 Genioglossus muscle visualized as VSP planned genioglossus-genioplasty osteotomy is advanced.

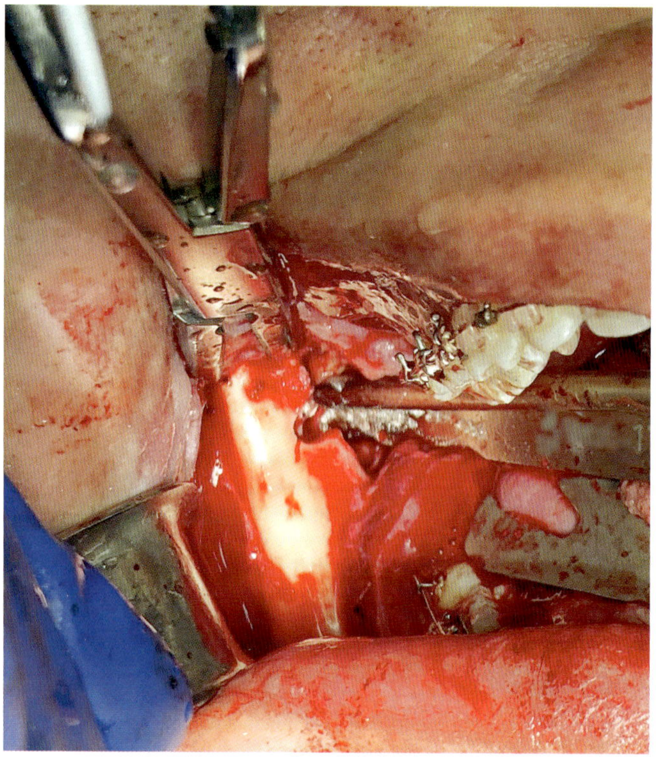

Fig. 12 Ramus medial exposure with groove.

visualization during the split to prevent uncontrolled fracture toward the condyle (Fig. 12).

14. Reciprocating saw is used to make the osteotomy, with the exception of the anterior osteotomy. The osteotomy needs to be long to ensure adequate bony overlap for fixation in large advancements (mandible usually advancing 12–15 mm measured at the pogonion). The anterior osteotomy is performed with a long-shank fissured bur to control the depth. The goal is to not overextend toward the lingual side. Classically described extension to the lingual side makes for an easy split but excessively thin bone on the posterior dentate segment for fixation.
15. Mandibular sagittal split begins with a full horizontal osteotomy to just past the lingula, followed by confirmation of osteotomy through the inferior border of mandible at the anterior, and the fragments are gently wedged open with osteotomes. No spreaders are used.
16. After final splint is applied with maxillomandibular fixation performed both around suspension wires and banded molar teeth, transfacial trocar approach is used for the first 2 or 3 positional screws. Mandibular plate is used to bridge what is usually a 1.2-cm to 2-cm gap (Figs. 13 and 14).
17. The final splint is removed to ensure stable occlusion without condylar sag and with bilateral canine guidance in excursive movement.
18. 3-0 Vicryl sutures are used to close the mandibular incisions. 3-0 chromic sutures are used for the V-Y cinch (where applicable) and maxillary incision.
19. Elastics are used in class 2 fashion in the molars but are kept light enough such that the patient can still breathe orally during the first week when nasal and sinus congestion is significant. Patients are not kept in a splint unless segmental osteotomies are absolutely required.

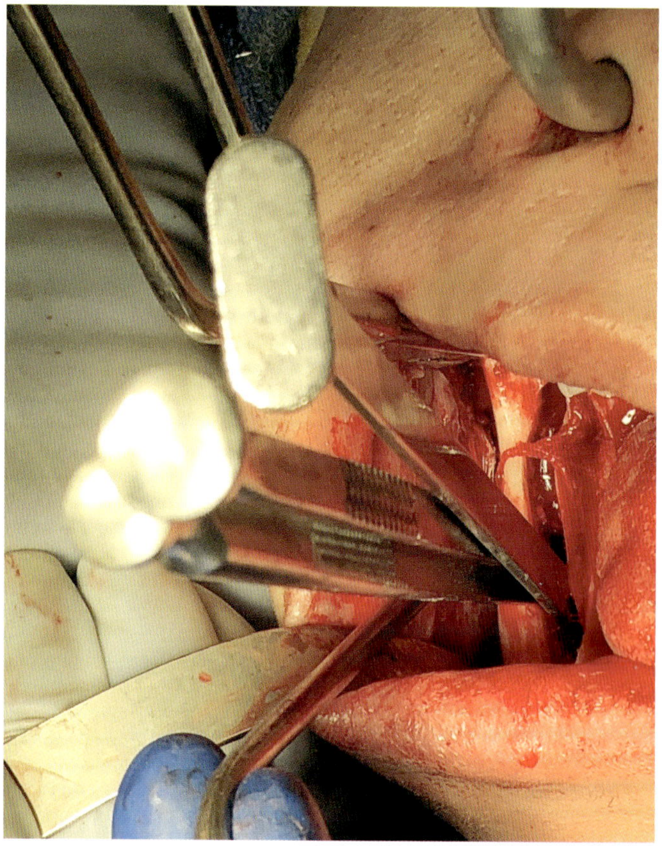

Fig. 13 Condylar and dentate segments wedged apart sequentially with three osteotomes.

Potential complications

The reported complication rate of MMA in literature is low.[12–14]

Intraoperative

During maxillary down-facture, injury to the descending palatine artery can occur. Care should be taken to remove bone associated with the palatine process of the maxilla to identify and preserve the neurovascular bundle. Although in the orthognathic literature it is well established that integrity of the descending palatine artery is not necessary, the authors have seen in older patients with severe OSA minor and temporary signs of inadequate perfusion. Hence, in general, the authors preserve the descending palatine arteries.

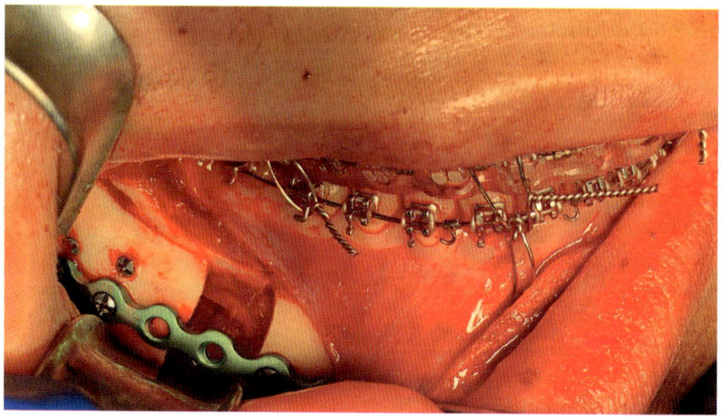

Fig. 14 Position screw and plate.

Ways to prevent buccal plate fracture or other types of uncontrolled split in OSA patients undergoing MMA have specifically been addressed in the surgical techniques section of this article.

Early postoperative

The most serious complication is airway obstruction, which should be acutely recognized. The authors' moderate to severe OSA patients spend the first evening in the ICU after extubation in the operating room. The authors do not band the jaws of post-MMA patients tightly nor place them in a splint. By not using a splint postoperatively and only using light guiding elastics, patients are allowed to orally breathe while congested and have easy access to suctioning when needed.

Malocclusion may occur as an early or late sequela of MMA surgery and may be correctable with orthodontics or requires revision surgery. Malocclusion with condylar sag can be addressed with repeat plating and careful attention paid to seating of the condylar segment.

Given the significant advancement, wound dehiscence is often seen at the site of mandibular incisions. Small dehiscence routinely closes with attentive clinical follow-up, washout, and home care instructions. Significant dehiscence with formulation of granulation tissue most often occurs over the area of dead space between the 2.4-mm mandibular plate and the mandibular advancement gap. Again, home care and washout are indicated, and hardware removal when the mandible is stable solves the problem.

Late postoperative

Malunion of the mandible can occur in the late postoperative period, necessitating bone grafting with a revision procedure. This is rare and can result from either a fracture or from inadequate fixation early on.

Hardware issues relating to chronic sinusitis, acute infection, or persistent pain secondary to maxillary and mandibular hardware are recognized in the orthognathic literature.[15,16] In the authors' population, hardware removal rate approaches 15%. Mandibular hardware is most commonly removed.

Relapse of the maxilla or mandible requires revision surgery. Depending on the degree of relapse, bone grafts from the symphysis (if no genioglossus advancement was performed) or the calvarium are good options.

Based on a review of more than 370 MMA patients from Stanford, approximately 18.7% underwent functional or esthetic nasal surgery approximately 1.5 years after surgery.[17] This rate has decreased to less than 5% in the recent 120 patients with judicious midfacial contouring and intraoperative septoplasty and inferior turbinate reduction with outfracture.

Clinical results in the literature

MMA consistently demonstrates high surgical success rate and moderate cure rate, and this is well described in several systematic review and a meta-analysis. A systematic review in 2010 performed by Holty and colleagues[1] described 627 adult patients with OSA across 22 diverse patient groups. They reported a mean apnea-hypopnea index (AHI) reduction from 63.9 to 9.5 events per hour. An update to this meta-analysis was performed by Zaghi and colleagues[5] in 2016, which included 518 patients across 45 studies. They reported success and cure rates of 85.5% and 38%, respectively. When compared with continuous positive airway pressure (CPAP), both Riley and Powell, of Stanford, and Vicini of Forli, Italy, independently showed MMA to be as effective based on the AHI and Epworth Sleepiness Scale in evidence level 2 and level 3 studies.[18,19]

Because the risk of cardiovascular comorbidity in severe OSA patients is much greater than that of healthy controls, MMA has shown to significantly reduce blood pressure.[20] This also has significant implications for the strong association between OSA and stroke.[21]

MMA compares favorably to CPAP with regard to improvement in sleep quality. Although the increase in rapid eye movement sleep is comparable between CPAP and MMA, MMA has shown additional decrease in wakefulness after sleep onset, a measure for sleep disturbance. A patient treated with MMA can restore sleep architecture comparable to a younger, healthy individual.[22]

Summary

MMA is one of the most defining operations for the treatment of OSA. It is characterized by predictably high success rate with low morbidity. The unique center of rotation for CCW movement maximizes skeletal advancement leading to airway stability. Proper contouring of the midface and intraoperative septoplasty maintain midfacial esthetics and improve nasal function. In the era of tissue-sparing palatopharyngoplasty, transoral robotic surgery, and upper airway stimulation of the hypoglossal nerve, MMA augmented by these interventions confers a higher chance of cure than ever in the history of sleep surgery.

Supplementary data

Supplementary data related to this article can be found online at https://doi.org/10.1016/j.cxom.2018.11.011.

References

1. Holty JE, Guilleminault C. Maxillomandibular advancement for the treatment of obstructive sleep apnea: a systematic review and meta-analysis. Sleep Med Rev 2010;14(5):287–97.
2. Liu SY, Huon LK, Iwasaki T, et al. Efficacy of maxillomandibular advancement examined with drug-induced sleep endoscopy and computational fluid dynamics airflow modeling. Otolaryngol Head Neck Surg 2016;154(1):189–95.
3. Prinsell JR. Maxillomandibular advancement surgery in a site-specific treatment approach for obstructive sleep apnea in 50 consecutive patients. Chest 1999;116(6):1519–29.
4. Riley RW, Powell NB, Guilleminault C. Maxillary, mandibular, and hyoid advancement for treatment of obstructive sleep apnea: a review of 40 patients. J Oral Maxillofac Surg 1990;48(1):20–6.
5. Zaghi S, Holty JE, Certal V, et al. Maxillomandibular advancement for treatment of obstructive sleep apnea: a meta-analysis. JAMA Otolaryngol Head Neck Surg 2016;142(1):58–66.
6. Riley RW, Powell NB. Maxillofacial surgery and obstructive sleep apnea syndrome. Otolaryngol Clin North Am 1990;23(4):809–26.
7. Riley RW, Powell NB, Guilleminault C. Obstructive sleep apnea syndrome: a surgical protocol for dynamic upper airway reconstruction. J Oral Maxillofac Surg 1993;51(7):742–7 [discussion: 748–9].

8. Liu SY, Huon LK, Lo MT, et al. Static craniofacial measurements and dynamic airway collapse patterns associated with severe obstructive sleep apnoea: a sleep MRI study. Clin Otolaryngol 2016;41(6):700–6.
9. Vanderveken OM, Maurer JT, Hohenhorst W, et al. Evaluation of drug-induced sleep endoscopy as a patient selection tool for implanted upper airway stimulation for obstructive sleep apnea. J Clin Sleep Med 2013;9(5):433–8.
10. Soares D, Sinawe H, Folbe AJ, et al. Lateral oropharyngeal wall and supraglottic airway collapse associated with failure in sleep apnea surgery. Laryngoscope 2012;122(2):473–9.
11. Yu CC, Bergeron L, Lin CH, et al. Single-splint technique in orthognathic surgery: intraoperative checkpoints to control facial symmetry. Plast Reconstr Surg 2009;124(3):879–86.
12. Blumen MB, Buchet I, Meulien P, et al. Complications/adverse effects of maxillomandibular advancement for the treatment of OSA in regard to outcome. Otolaryngol Head Neck Surg 2009;141(5):591–7.
13. Camacho M, Liu SY, Certal V, et al. Large maxillomandibular advancements for obstructive sleep apnea: an operative technique evolved over 30 years. J Craniomaxillofac Surg 2015;43(7):1113–8.
14. Li KK, Riley R, Powell N. Complications of obstructive sleep apnea surgery. Oral Maxillofac Surg Clin North Am 2003;15(2):297–304.
15. Falter B, Schepers S, Vrielinck L, et al. Plate removal following orthognathic surgery. Oral Surg Oral Med Oral Pathol Oral Radiol Endod 2011;112(6):737–43.
16. Schmidt BL, Perrott DH, Mahan D, et al. The removal of plates and screws after Le Fort I osteotomy. J Oral Maxillofac Surg 1998;56(2):184–8.
17. Liu SY, Lee PJ, Awad M, et al. Corrective nasal surgery after maxillomandibular advancement for obstructive sleep apnea: experience from 379 cases. Otolaryngol Head Neck Surg 2017; 157(1):156–9.
18. Riley RW, Powell NB, Guilleminault C. Maxillofacial surgery and nasal CPAP. A comparison of treatment for obstructive sleep apnea syndrome. Chest 1990;98(6):1421–5.
19. Vicini C, Dallan I, Campanini A, et al. Surgery vs ventilation in adult severe obstructive sleep apnea syndrome. Am J Otolaryngol 2010; 31(1):14–20.
20. Islam S, Taylor CJ, Ormiston IW. Effects of maxillomandibular advancement on systemic blood pressure in patients with obstructive sleep apnoea. Br J Oral Maxillofac Surg 2015;53(1): 34–8.
21. Yaggi HK, Concato J, Kernan WN, et al. Obstructive sleep apnea as a risk factor for stroke and death. N Engl J Med 2005;353(19): 2034–41.
22. Liu SY, Huon LK, Ruoff C, et al. Restoration of sleep architecture after maxillomandibular advancement: success beyond the apnea-hypopnea index. Int J Oral Maxillofac Surg 2017;46(12):1533–8.

Further readings

Liu SY, Huon LK, Powell NB, et al. Lateral pharyngeal wall tension after maxillomandibular advancement for obstructive sleep apnea is a marker for surgical success: observations from drug-induced sleep endoscopy. J Oral Maxillofac Surg 2015;73(8): 1575–82.

Prinsell JR. Primary and secondary telegnathic maxillomandibular advancement, with or without adjunctive procedures, for obstructive sleep apnea in adults: a literature review and treatment recommendations. J Oral Maxillofac Surg 2012;70(7):1659–77.

Riley RW, Powell NB, Guilleminault C. Obstructive sleep apnea syndrome: a review of 306 consecutively treated surgical patients. Otolaryngol Head Neck Surg 1993;108(2):117–25.

Waite PD, Wooten V, Lachner J, et al. Maxillomandibular advancement surgery in 23 patients with obstructive sleep apnea syndrome. J Oral Maxillofac Surg 1989;47(12):1256–61 [discussion: 1262].

Maxillomandibular Advancement

The Canadian Experience

Mélinda Paris, DMD, MSc, FRCDC*, Simon Jean, DMD ,
Carl Bouchard, DMD, MSc, FRCDC

KEYWORDS

• Maxillofacial surgery • Orthognathic surgery • Obstructive sleep apnea • Maxillomandibular advancement

KEY POINTS

- Obstructive sleep apnea is underdiagnosed in Canada.
- Canadian sleep specialists are reluctant to propose maxillomandibular advancement (MMA).
- The Canadian public health insurance covers expenses related to sleep apnea investigation and MMA (with the exception of orthodontic treatment).
- MMA treatment plan is based on a multiple of factors, such as obstructive sleep apnea severity, aesthetics, and the initial malocclusion.

Introduction

Obstructive sleep apnea (OSA) is a chronic medical condition characterized by a temporary reduction or a cessation of airflow. It is acknowledged that continuous positive airway pressure (CPAP) is the first line of treatment, but, like most patients affected by this disease, Canadians are looking for a definitive cure. Maxillomandibular advancement (MMA) is an effective surgical treatment that is nowadays more frequently proposed to the Canadian population, although there is still a general lack of knowledge among sleep specialists on its indications and efficacy. Similarly, general dentists tend to favor dental mandibular advancement devices (DMADs) because they are more familiar with them. The goal of this article is to expose the authors' experience with MMA for the treatment of this condition.

An estimated 5.4 million Canadians have been diagnosed with OSA or at risk of developing it.[1] In 2009, based on a questionnaire survey sent to 8647 adults, the Canadian Public Health Agency estimated that approximately 858,900 Canadians adults were diagnosed with OSA by their physician[1]; 75% of these patients were older than 45 years old.[1] The study also reported that 26% of the Canadian population is at risk of developing OSA in the near future based on risk factors and symptoms of OSA.[1]

The Canadian population is more aware of OSA, and referral to sleep clinics has increased in the recent years.[2] The public health survey estimated that 76% of Canadians diagnosed with OSA and 4.8% of patients considered at high risk of OSA were referred for a sleep apnea investigation.[1] OSA diagnosis in Canada seems to be made by doctors without a polysomnographic study.[1,2] Access to a polysomnographic examination represents a challenge in many centers, and this may explain why 23% of patients who reported symptoms of OSA never had this test.[1] Evans and colleagues[2] published a study showing that the amount of sleep laboratories in the country is approximately 2 per 100,000 population.

Because patients living in rural areas have less access to these facilities, they are more likely to be undiagnosed and have more severe disease at time of diagnosis.[3,4]

The Canadian health care system

In Canada, the health care system is public and OSA treatments are generally insured. This may vary slightly between provinces (10) and territories (3) because both are responsible for delivering health services.[3] One possible drawback of this system is an increased waiting period to meet sleep specialists and to obtain appropriate diagnosis and treatment. This may be one of the reasons why the number of private sleep clinics has increased in the past decade.[2] CPAP appliances and DMADs are usually at a patient's expense. This is also the case for orthodontics even if it is judged necessary to proceed to MMA.

The dental community is biased toward the use of DMADs, and sleep physicians are reluctant to refer patients for MMA. The benefits and efficacy of MMA still need to be promoted as it is often considered as too invasive and risky by other sleep specialists. Results obtained with MMA in Canadian centers have been published, showing good clinical results.[5–8]

Disclosure Statement: The authors have nothing to disclose.

Service de chirurgie buccale et maxillo-faciale, CHU de Québec-Université Laval, Hôpital de l'Enfant-Jésus, 1401 18e rue, Québec city, Québec G1J 1Z4, Canada

* Corresponding author.

E-mail address: melinda.paris.1@ulaval.ca

Atlas Oral Maxillofacial Surg Clin N Am 27 (2019) 37-42

https://doi.org/10.1016/j.cxom.2018.11.007

The CHU de Québec-Université Laval-Hôpital de l'Enfant-Jésus experience and surgical technique

The authors' academic institution performs more than 300 cases of standard orthognathic surgery per year. Referrals for MMA for OSA patients are increasing. Otorhinolaryngologists, pneumologists, family doctors, and dentists refer most OSA patients. At the authors' institution, before considering MMA, all patients need a confirmed OSA diagnosis with polysomnography. A trial period of CPAP therapy is also strongly recommended unless obvious craniofacial anomalies are noted (Fig. 1). If a patient has a dental malocclusion or a retrusive facial profile, a consultation with an orthodontist is recommended to decompensate the occlusion and allow more forward movement of the maxillomandibular complex. On the other hand, MMA may be accomplished without an orthodontic preparation.

Preoperative planning

Once a patient is considered a good candidate for MMA, the following data are recorded: cephalometric and panoramic radiographs, CT, full facial photographs, dental impressions, and all other relevant clinical information. Maxillofacial orthognathic treatment plan is based on several factors. The aesthetics outcome related to MMA is explained to the patient. Negative aesthetics effects are possible but rare with low effect if the surgery is well planned.[6,8]

For bimaxillary surgery, a counterclockwise rotation of the maxillomandibular complex is often planned to maximize the mandibular advancement to open the posterior airway and diminish collapsibility. The amount of advancement and rotation is based on the patient malocclusion, appearance, and OSA severity. The first goal is to correct the OSA by enhancing the airway and to correct the malocclusion by maintaining an aesthetic normal facial balance and a stable dental occlusion, although it is important to consider the patient facial appearance to minimize the negative effect of this approach. A patient with thick soft tissue tolerates an anticlockwise rotation and a large maxillary advancement better aesthetically than a patient with thin facial soft tissue. A patient with solely retrognathic mandible with an orthognathic maxilla and moderate OSA may benefit merely of a bilateral sagittal split osteotomy (BSSO) advancement with genioplasty only. Research has shown that a sole BSSO brings tridimensional volumetric changes in the airway by enlarging the airway space when a retrusive mandible is present.[9–11]

Cephalometric radiograph is traced with the architectural and structural Delaire analysis.[5,7,12,13] Delaire cephalometric analysis is based on skeletal points.[12] Delaire analysis uses the nasopalatine canal and the menton region to determine mandible and maxillary positions.[12] Those skeletal landmarks are less influenced by the dentoalveolar area of the patient, such as A and B points, and are proved to correlate the severity of apnea-hypopnea index (AHI) with the bimaxillary sagittal position with more efficacies.[12] The authors use virtual surgical planning for all cases. This surgical planning allows analyzing the bony modification and future bimaxillary position more precisely. Both condyles are specifically placed in the posterior glenoid fossa.

For OSA patients treated by their orthodontist with multibracket appliances or clear aligners, surgical hooks or orthodontic brackets are installed prior to the surgery date.

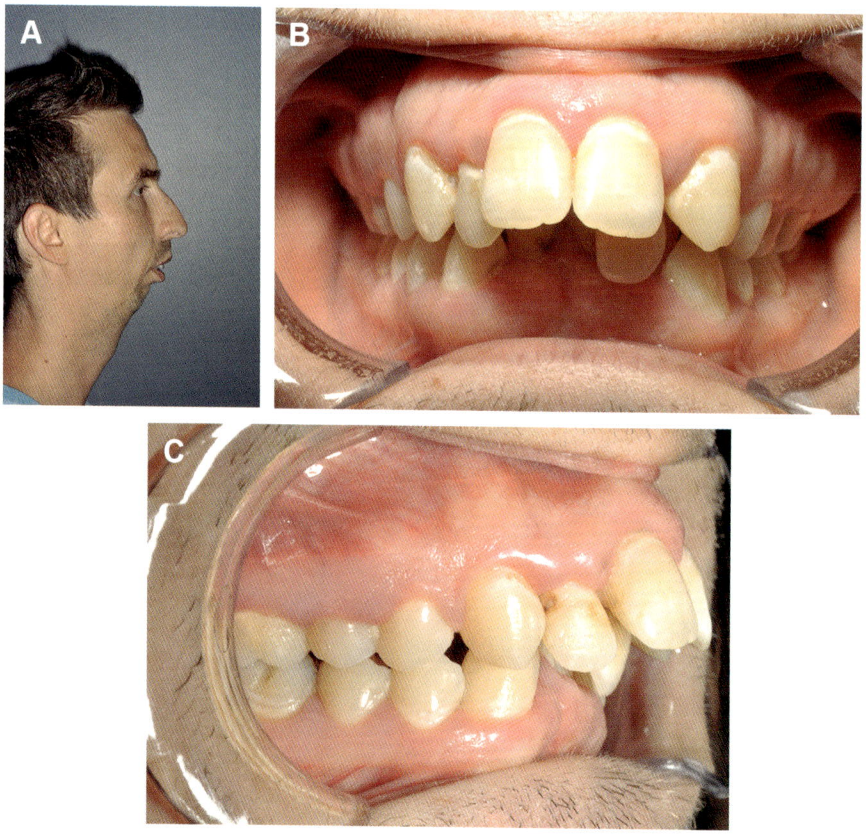

Fig. 1 *A*) Facial and (*B*, *C*) intraoral pictures of a 28-year-old male patient with severe retrognathia.

Patient preparation

Patients are placed in supine position and put under general anesthesia with nasotracheal intubation. A nasogastric tube and arterial line are installed for all patients. Local anesthesia of the mucosa and inferior alveolar nerve blocs are performed using bupivacaine 0.5% with epinephrine 1:200,000 for postoperative anesthesia. Occlusal adjustments of the teeth are done when necessary at this point. For patients without active orthodontic treatment, temporary dental brackets or intermaxillary fixation (IMF) screws are installed for intraoperative IMF and postoperative guiding elastics when judged necessary. Otherwise the screws are removed at the end of surgery.

Surgical technique and approaches

The authors generally preconized a mandible-first sequence for OSA patients to obtain a more stable intermediate position; otherwise, the splint is too large and IMF is more difficult to place.

For the BSSO approach, bilateral vestibular incision is realized. Full subperiosteal dissection is performed and the lingula is identified. All ostectomies are performed using a combination of reciprocating saw and Lindemann bur. Splitting of the mandible according to the osteotomies is completed with osteotomes and bone spreaders. The inferior alveolar nerve is identified and bone interferences are removed.

The intermediate guiding splint is installed and patient is placed in IMF. The authors carefully adapt the proximal to the distal bone segment by grinding bone interferences with a surgical rasp. This is particularly important if fixation with bicortical screws is contemplated. Titanium mandibular rigid fixation is applied with either bicortical screws, titanium plates, or a combination of both (Fig. 2). With mandibular advancement, the airway is then opened by advancement of the suprahyoid muscles, the anterior digastrics, and the mylohyoid muscles.[5] IMF is released and the intermediate position is confirmed. Attention can then be on the maxilla.

For the maxilla, unisegmental or multisegmental Le Fort I osteotomy is planned depending on the need for maxillary expansion. With maxillary transverse expansion, the airway and the nasal floor are then enlarged and the nasal airway resistance is reduced, which may help cure OSA. Maxillary and mandibular transverse expansions are, in rare cases, recommended (Fig. 3). The authors do not bone graft most of the maxilla, but, if judged necessary (larger advancement, thin maxillary bone, bruxism, or surgeon preference), the anterior iliac crest is generally preferred.

The authors use a Kirschner (K)-wire at nasion as an external vertical guide for positioning the maxilla. Bilateral vestibular incisions are realized with electrocautery. The entire maxilla is skeletonized up to the infraorbital nerves and posteriorly to pterygomaxillary fissure. The nasal mucosa is detached from the maxilla and standard horizontal cuts are done with a reciprocating saw while protecting nasal mucosa and buccal soft tissues with malleable retractors. Osteotomies are completed to the pterygoid plates with a spatula osteotome. The lateral nasal wall is also osteotomized with this instrument. The nasal septum osteotomy and pterygomaxillary disjunction are completed with their respective osteotomes. Controlled hypotensive anesthesia is executed and confirmed with the arterial cannula. The maxilla is then down-fractured and mobilized with Rowe forceps. Potential bony interferences, especially posteriorly, are removed. Inferior turbinate reduction or septoplasty may be realized as needed to prevent deviation and to increase nasal airway. The final guiding splint is installed and patient is placed in IMF. Vertical position of the maxilla is confirmed with the K-wire. When vertical position is judged satisfactory, titanium plates are applied on piriform and malar rims (Fig. 4). The IMF is released and the final occlusion is verified.

The authors follow with a precise shaving of the anterior maxillary region with the objective of minimizing the

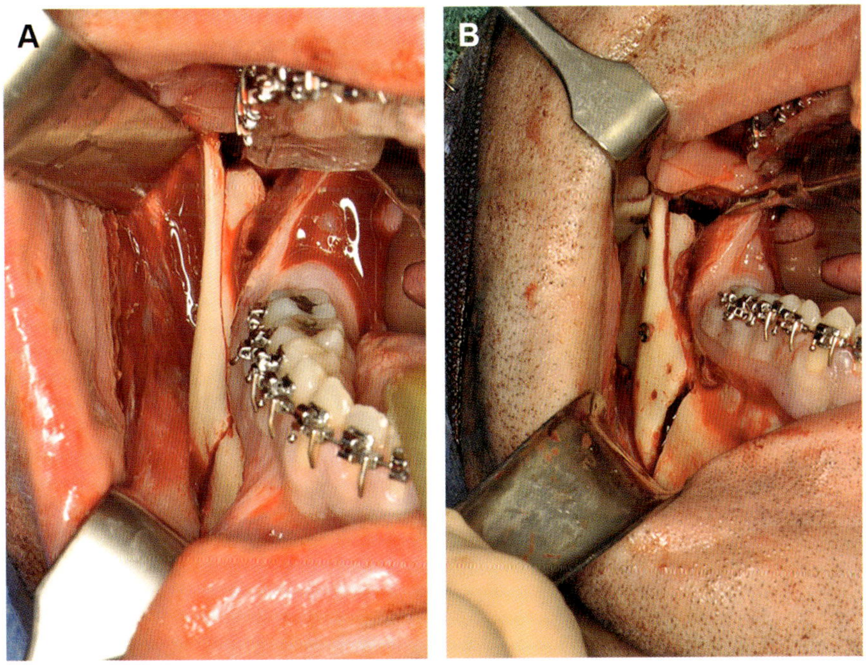

Fig. 2 Mandibular osteotomies are performed with a reciprocating saw and Lindemann bur (*A*). Bicortical screws are used for fixation (*B*).

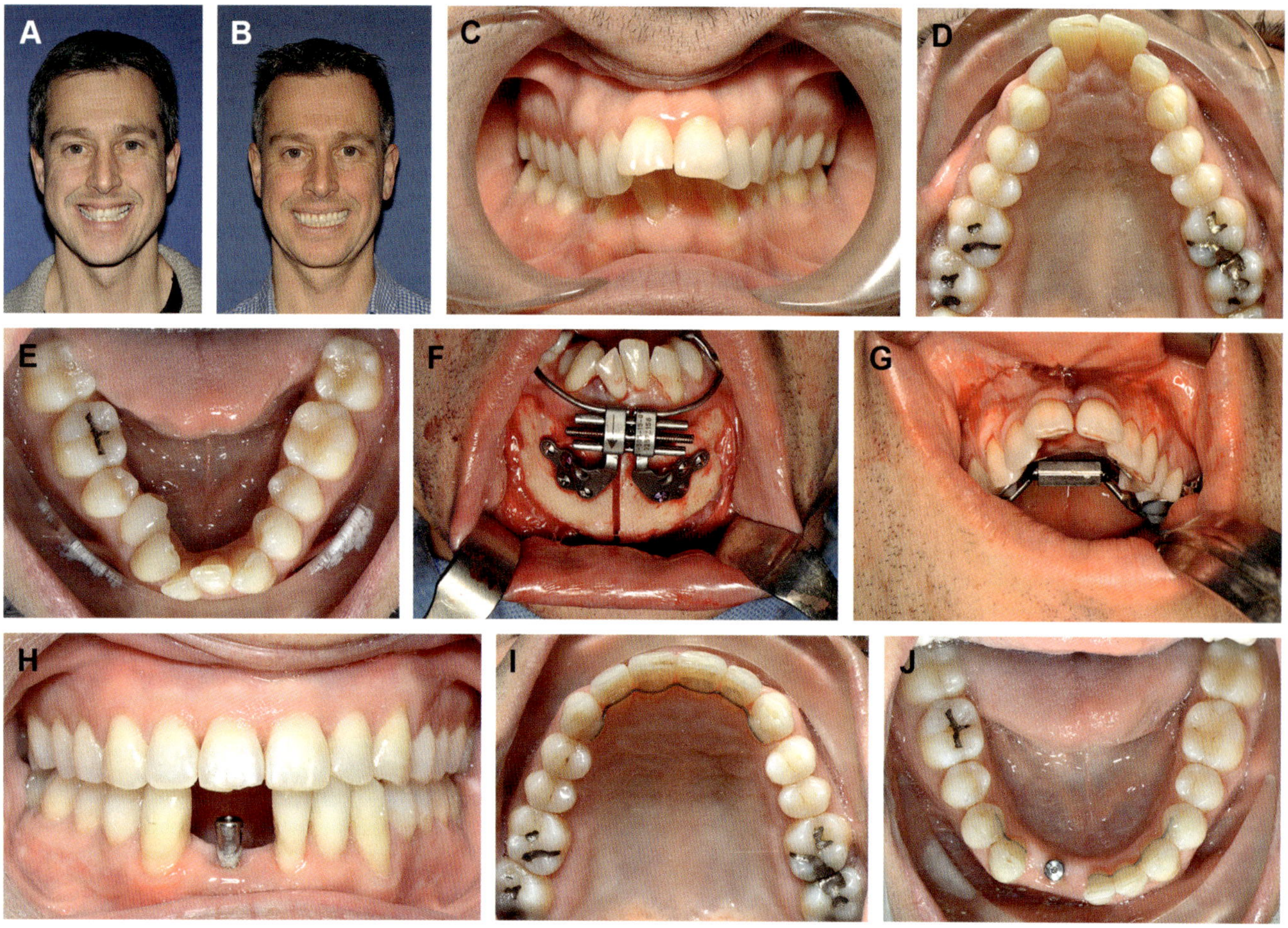

Fig. 3 Frontal preoperative (*A*) and postoperative (*B*) photographs of a 43-year-old male patient with severe constriction of the maxilla (*C*, *D*) and mandible (*E*) treated by transverse expansion of both maxilla (*F*, *G*). Postoperative dental photographs (*H–J*). The patient is now completely asymptomatic from his sleep disorder disease. ([E-I-J] Courtesy of Dr Sylvain Chamberland, DMD, Quebec city, Canada.)

potentially negative aesthetic effect of a major maxillary advancement on the nasal region and soft tissue. The anterior nasal spine, the external nasal cavities, the piriform region, and the midline alveolar region are recontoured with a surgical bur.

Whenever possible from an aesthetic point of view, a genioplasty is realized to increase treatment success. Conventional (Fig. 5), tenon, and mortise (Fig. 6) or genial tubercle genioplasty (Fig. 7) are performed when judged appropriate.

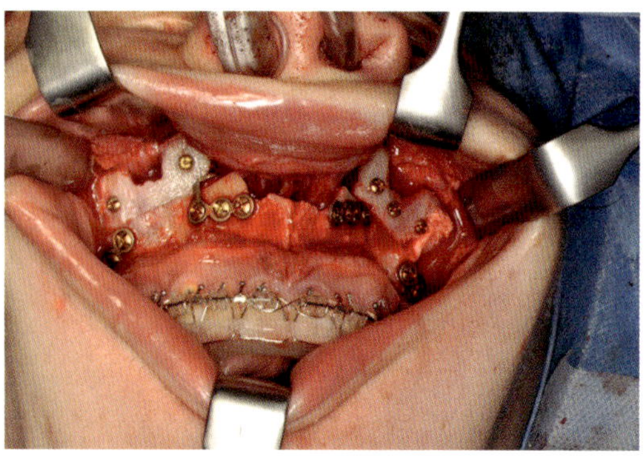

Fig. 4 Conventional Le Fort I osteotomy after rigid internal fixation. Bone harvested from the anterior iliac crest were grafted to fill bone gap.

All sites are thoroughly irrigated with a saline solution. The nasal septum if attached to the anterior nasal spine with polyglactin 910 sutures (Vicryl, Ethicon, Somerville, New Jersey). The same type of suture is used for the transnasal cinch suture and mental muscles. The authors use 3-0 and 4-0 Chromic Gut (Ethicon, Somerville, New Jersey) for mucosal closure.

Immediate postoperative care

Patients are placed on 2 to 4 guiding elastics when judged appropriate. Those elastics are placed on temporary dental

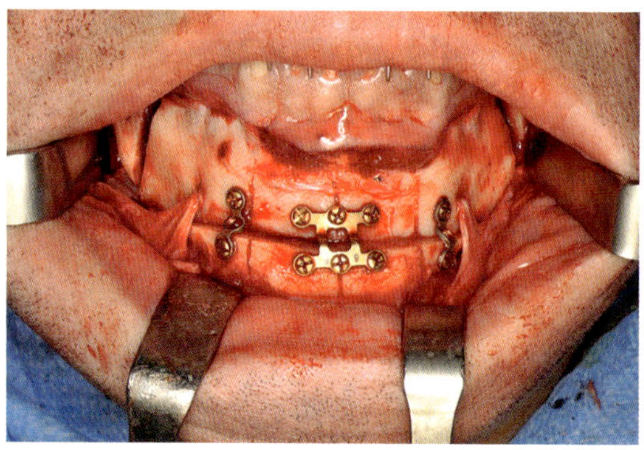

Fig. 5 Conventional genioplasty.

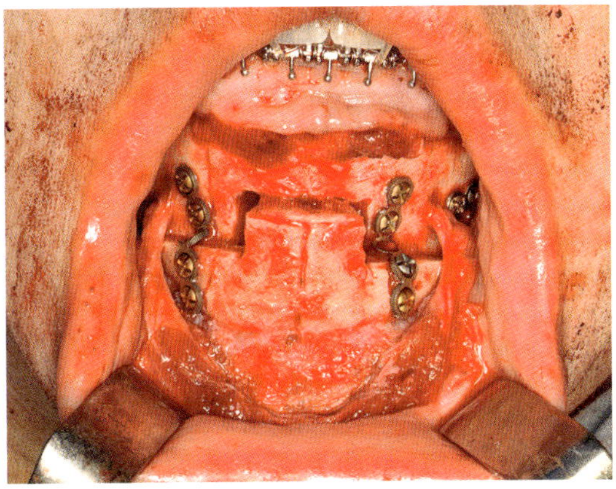

Fig. 6 Tenons and mortise genioplasty designed to ensure that the genial tubercles are advanced.

brackets, surgical post, or fixation screws. If a patient is treated with clear aligners, their need to wear their aligners to be placed under guiding elastics or dental extrusion may occur.

Postoperative care is conventional as for any orthognathic surgery cases. Immediately after surgery, patients are extubated and monitored on the surgical floor. No intensive care is needed. Rapid patient mobilization and hydration are mandatory. The patient is discharged at postoperative day 1 or day 2 depending on recovery. Patients are placed on a soft diet for 2 weeks. Many patients report a better sleep quality even at postoperative day 1. A postoperative polysomnography is prescribed 6 months after surgery to compare their AHI and evaluate their residual or cure of OSA.

Potential complications

Complications after MMA advancement are relatively similar to those for conventional MMA. Hypoesthesia of the second and third trigeminal branches are possible. Infection, edema, malunion, and reintervention procedures are complications that are possible. Patients treated with MMA to cure their OSA, however, do not present more risk for those complications. Considering that the mandible is advancing more anteriorly, a posterior mandibular relapse may occur.

Discussion of these complications is mandatory during the preoperative discussion. The AHI index may not be correct and OSA symptoms may remain present. Patients may still need to wear their CPAP. Negative aesthetics outcomes may appear and the patient may be unsatisfied with the aesthetic outcome.

Results

The authors conducted a retrospective study based on a hospital chart revision from January 2012 to June 2017. Nine oral and maxillofacial staff surgeons operated on this retrospective cohort of patients. Throughout this time, 67 patients underwent an orthognathic surgery procedure for OSA. The hospital charts of all 67 patients were reviewed by one of the authors (Dr Jean). Patients' mean age was 46 years old, ranging from 19 years to 73 years old: 48 patients were men and 19 were women; 9 patients had mild preoperative OSA; 23 had moderate OSA; and 21 were classified as having severe OSA. The initial AHI could not be tracked down for 14 patients; 41 patients had MMA with concomitant advancement genioplasty. Forward movement of the maxilla ranged from 2 mm to 12 mm, 7 mm to 13.5 mm for the mandible, and 4 mm to 10 mm for the chin.

Postoperative polysomnography reports were available for 25 of the 67 patients (Table 1). These results showed surgical success in 8 patients (32%) (AHI <20 and 50% reduction in AHI) or a cure in 9 patients (36%) (AHI <5). The authors' overall therapeutic success for OSA patients undergoing an MMA procedure was 68% (17/25 patients). AHI was not significantly improved in 8 patients (32%). Of these 8 patients, 2 had

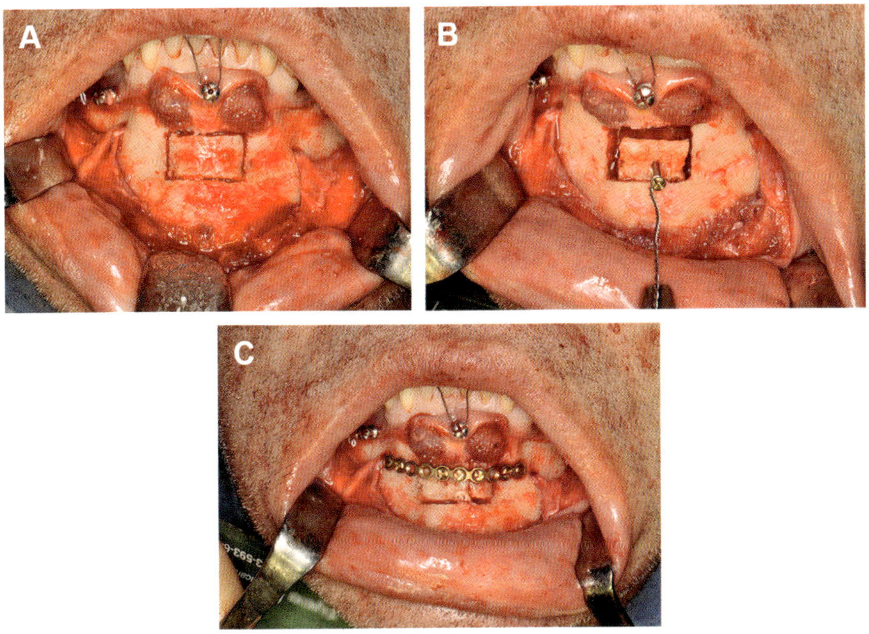

Fig. 7 Genial tubercle advancement genioplasty. The outer bone cortex of the chin is cut and removed with sufficient length and width to grasp genial tubercles (*A*). It is then moved forward (*B*) and plated to the outer cortical bone (*C*).

Table 1 Descriptive statistics of patient with preoperative and postoperative polysomnography after orthognathic treatment

Study Variables	Descriptive Statistics
Sample size (n patients)	25
Gender	
Male	14 (56%)
Female	11 (44%)
Ages ±SD	49.3 ± 9.9 (30–73)
Procedure	
MMA	9 (36%)
MMA + genioplasty	16 (64%)
Preoperative OSA	
Mild	3 (12%)
Moderate	11 (44%)
Severe	11 (44%)
Postoperative OSA	
Mild	19 (76%)
Moderate	6 (24%)
Severe	0
Surgical success	8 (32%)
Surgical cure	9 (36%)
Nonsignificant improvement	8 (32%)
Overall therapeutic success	17 (68%)

preoperative mild OSA, 4 had preoperative moderate OSA, and 2 had preoperative severe OSA. The results obtained in this series (68% surgical success) are lower than what was reported in a recent meta-analysis (85.5% surgical success).[14] This could be explained by the fact that 42 of 67 patients (63%) did not return for postoperative polysomnographic evaluation, assuming that patients with a positive outcome are less likely to undergo further examination.

Postoperative polysomnography results could not be obtained for all patients with OSA who underwent MMA in the authors' center. Subjective data, however, which were discussed through follow-up appointments, could be retrieved in hospital charts; 4 patients stated that their snoring completely ceased postoperatively; 4 patients stopped using their CPAP equipment after the orthognathic surgery because they were either more energetic in their daily life or they had a more recuperative sleep; and 1 of these 4 patients had an unexpected postoperative AHI increase from 15 to 23 episodes per hour but still discontinued CPAP therapy because of favorable subjective outcomes. Two patients who had a preoperative severe OSA still use their CPAP equipment because they are symptomatic. One of these 2 patients had a reduction of AHI from 31 to 15 episodes per hour but is as symptomatic as in his preoperative state.

OSA is a disease known worldwide. Medical professions are more aware of this condition. Oral and maxillofacial surgeons play a significant role in the diagnosis, treatment plan, and cure of OSA. Treatment plan of MMA is a cornerstone in the authors' practice.

References

1. Public Health Agency of Canada. What is the impact of sleep apnea on Canadians? Her Majesty the Queen in Right of Canada 2010:1–3.
2. Evans J, Skomro R, Driver H, et al. Sleep laboratory test referrals in Canada: sleep apnea rapid response survey. Can Respir J 2014; 21(1):e4–10.
3. Pendharkar SR, Povitz M, Bansback N, et al. Testing and treatment for obstructive sleep apnea in Canada: funding models must change. CMAJ 2017;189(49):E1524–8.
4. Allen AJ, Amram O, Tavakoli H, et al. Relationship between travel time from home to a regional sleep apnea Clinic in British Columbia, Canada, and the severity of obstructive sleep. Ann Am Thorac Soc 2016;13(5):719–23.
5. Goodday R. Diagnosis, treatment planning, and surgical correction of obstructive sleep apnea. J Oral Maxillofac Surg 2009;67(10): 2183–96.
6. Goodday R, Bourque S. Subjective outcomes of maxillomandibular advancement surgery for treatment of obstructive sleep apnea syndrome. J Oral Maxillofac Surg 2012;70(2):417–20.
7. Goodday RH, Bourque SE, Edwards PB. Objective and subjective outcomes following maxillomandibular advancement surgery for treatment of patients with extremely severe obstructive sleep apnea (apnea-hypopnea index >100). J Oral Maxillofac Surg 2016; 74(3):583–9.
8. Curran J. Aesthetic outcome of maxillomandibular advancement surgery for the treatment of obstructive sleep apnea. London (Canada): Western University Graduate & POstdoctoral Studies, Western University; 2017.
9. Ristow O, Ruckschloss T, Berger M, et al. Short- and long-term changes of the pharyngeal airway after surgical mandibular advancement in Class II patients-a three-dimensional retrospective study. J Craniomaxillofac Surg 2018;46(1):56–62.
10. Noller MW, Guilleminault C, Gouveia CJ, et al. Mandibular advancement for adult obstructive sleep apnea: a systematic review and meta-analysis. J Craniomaxillofac Surg 2017;45(12): 2035–40.
11. De Oliveira DL, Calcagnotto T, Vago TM, et al. Tomographic analysis of the impact of mandibular advancement surgery on increased airway volume. Ann Maxillofac Surg 2017;7(2):256–9.
12. Vezina JP, Blumen M, Buchet I, et al. Sleep-disordered breathing: choosing the right cephalometric analysis. J Oral Maxillofac Surg 2012;70(6):1442–8.
13. Delaire J. Pathogenic situations after orthodontic treatment. Defects in skeleton and soft tissues that should be avoided after orthodontic treatment. Orthod Fr 2011;82(4):359–66 [in French].
14. Zaghi S, Holty JE, Certal V, et al. Maxillomandibular advancement for treatment of obstructive sleep apnea: a meta-analysis. JAMA Otolaryngol Head Neck Surg 2016;142(1):58–66.

Bilateral Temporomandibular Joint Reconstruction and Maxillomandibular Advancement for Concomitant Temporomandibular Joint Degeneration and Obstructive Sleep Apnea

Rishi Jay Gupta, DDS, MD, MBA [a,b,c,*], Rebeka Silva, DMD, FACD [a,b], Stephen T. Connelly, DDS, MD, PhD [a,b]

KEYWORDS

- Temporomandibular disorder (TMD) • Obstructive sleep apnea (OSA) • Maxillomandibular advancement (MMA)
- Temporomandibular joint reconstruction (TJR)
- Maxillomandibular advancement with concomitant temporomandibular joint reconstruction • Virtual surgical planning (VSP)

KEY POINTS

- Association between temporomandibular disorder (TMD) and sleep disturbances, including obstructive sleep apnea (OSA), is well documented, although the underlying mechanisms remain unclear.
- Comprehensive diagnostic workup is critical in determining the appropriate selection of surgical options for patients with both OSA and TMD.
- Patients with TMD and OSA who are intolerant of medical therapies can be treated effectively with custom temporomandibular joint (TMJ) reconstruction in combination with maxillomandibular advancement (MMA).
- Virtual surgical planning is an accurate method to optimize MMA movements in setting of TMJ reconstruction.
- A detailed step-by-step protocol is essential to minimize intraoperative complications.

Introduction

Obstructive sleep apnea (OSA) is characterized by repeated collapse of the upper airway and cessation of breathing that leads to arousals and results in comorbidities, such as hypertension, stroke, myocardial infarction, and diabetes.[1,2] OSA has emerged as a medical condition that has considerable health and social repercussions. Temporomandibular joint (TMJ) disorders, such as degenerative joint disease, are characterized by pain and joint dysfunction that can lead to progressive condylar resorption and mandibular retrognathia, resulting in a malocclusion with anterior open bite and airway compromise. The association between temporomandibular disorder (TMD) and sleep disturbances, including OSA, is well documented, although the underlying mechanisms remain unclear.[3–5]

Patients with OSA who are intolerant of positive airway pressure therapy can be treated with maxillomandibular advancement (MMA) with high success rates.[6,7] However, there is a subset of OSA patients who also present with TMD that needs to be addressed to provide a stable and predictable outcome. Temporomandibular joint reconstruction (TJR) using custom prostheses in conjunction with orthognathic surgery has been used to treat TMD and craniofacial anomalies.[8–10] Bilateral TJR with concomitant MMA surgery is the solution that allows surgeons to treat both TMD and OSA simultaneously.[10–13]

The surgeon needs to have a thorough understanding of the preoperative and surgical protocols in order to enable efficiency, limit operative time, and deliver optimal postoperative outcomes. This article describes the steps required for preoperative assessment, virtual surgical planning (VSP), and performance of the bilateral TMJ reconstruction with MMA to treat TMD and OSA concurrently.

Disclosure Statement: The authors have nothing to disclose.

[a] Oral and Maxillofacial Surgery Section, Department of Dental Service, San Francisco VA Health Care System, 4150 Clement Street (160), San Francisco, CA 94121, USA

[b] Department of Oral and Maxillofacial Surgery, University of California, San Francisco, 707 Parnassus Ave, San Francisco, CA 94143, USA

[c] Department of Otolaryngology Head and Neck Surgery, University of California, Davis, 2521 Stockton Blvd, Sacramento, CA 95817, USA

* Corresponding author. Oral and Maxillofacial Surgery Section, Dental Service, San Francisco VA Health Care System, 4150 Clement Street (160), San Francisco, CA 94121.

E-mail address: rishi.gupta@va.gov

Atlas Oral Maxillofacial Surg Clin N Am 27 (2019) 43-52
1061-3315/19/Published by Elsevier Inc.
https://doi.org/10.1016/j.cxom.2018.11.006

Surgical technique

Diagnostic workup

A comprehensive diagnostic workup is critical in determining the appropriate selection of surgical options for patients with both OSA and TMD. The severity of pathologic condition associated with OSA and TMD will determine whether both pathologic conditions need to be surgically treated concomitantly versus one treated medically and the other surgically. Conservative medical treatment is always initiated first for each disorder. If conservative treatment allows for resolution of symptoms and stabilization of one of the pathologic conditions, then the other can be solely addressed surgically. Therefore, it is important to look at each disease as separate entities and also as synergistic processes. Indications for concomitant TJR and MMA include moderate to severe OSA and TMJ disorders, such as articular disc displacement, condylar resorption, ankylosis, congenital malformation, and arthritic changes.

Obstructive sleep apnea

Patients require a thorough clinical examination of the nasal passages, oropharyngeal space, and retroglossal area, taking note of the nasal septum, turbinates, uvula, soft palate, tonsils, tongue size and positioning, occlusal classification, and relative positioning of the maxilla and mandible. A baseline polysomnography (PSG) or home sleep study is needed to characterize the severity of the OSA according to the standards of the American Academy of Sleep Medicine. Radiographic evaluation of the airway includes a computed tomographic (CT) scan and lateral cephalometric analysis. A choke point of less than 50 mm^2 is associated with severe OSA, and greater than 150 mm^2 is generally normal.[14] Drug-induced sleep endoscopy (DISE) is a tool to identify areas of collapse and patterns of obstruction along the airway while the patient is asleep. DISE provides data to develop an accurate diagnosis and prescribe specific surgical treatments[15] targeted to correct the anatomic problem areas. The pattern and degree of collapse are scored according to the VOTE (velum, oropharyngeal, tongue base, and epiglottis) classification.[16,17]

Temporomandibular joint disorder

Patients require a detailed assessment of the functionality of the TMJ region, which includes palpation of the muscles of mastication and condyle, auscultation of the TMJ for clicking, popping, and crepitus, measuring the range of motion including maximum incisal opening, lateral excursive movements, deviation on opening and closing, and occlusal classification and stability. Radiographic evaluation includes a CT scan to look at joint space and condylar degenerative changes and an MRI to look for joint effusions and disc integrity and position in the open and closed mouth position.

These various diagnostic modalities should be used together to provide a comprehensive airway and TMJ evaluation to select an appropriate surgical treatment option.

Preoperative planning

Preoperative planning steps use virtual surgical technology. The custom, patient-specific TMJ prostheses are manufactured by TMJ Concepts (Ventura, CA, USA).

1. CT scan and dental casts sent with bite registration to the VSP company of choice (Fig. 1)
2. Models scanned and incorporated into CT scan
3. Virtual removal of condyles and ramus
4. Computer-aided planning session for final positioning of the maxilla and mandible with mandible surgery as the first approach (Fig. 2)
5. Final approval of jaw positions: VSP company fabricates intermediate and final splints
6. Finalized virtual planning data sent to TMJ Concepts
7. Stereolithic model constructed with jaws in final position, and TMJ Concepts performs design and wax-up of TMJ prostheses
8. Images of TMJ design and wax-up sent to surgeon for approval (Fig. 3)
9. TMJ Concepts manufactures custom fossa and condylar prostheses (Fig. 4)
10. Stereolithic model and TMJ prostheses (TMJ Concepts) and splints with dental models (VSP company) are sent to surgeon (Fig. 5)

Preparation and patient positioning

The patient is taken to the operating room, placed in the supine position, and intubated nasally. If orthodontic brackets and bands were not applied preoperatively, then traditional Erich or hybrid arch bars are placed. Bilateral Nerve Integrity Monitoring System probes (Medtronic, Minneapolis, MN, USA) are placed to monitor the branches of the facial nerve (Fig. 6). The external auditory canals are irrigated with around 300 ml of a 1:1 ratio of betadine and saline. The face and abdomen are then prepared with betadine and isolated with sterile towels and split sheet (Fig. 7). The mouth is isolated with Tegaderm (3M, St. Paul, MN, USA); gauze impregnated with petroleum jelly is placed in each ear canal, and the tragus is sutured closed. Then, 1010 drapes (3M) are placed to further isolate the oral cavity from the surgical field. The patient is given decadron and intravenous (IV) antibiotics before the start of the surgical procedure.

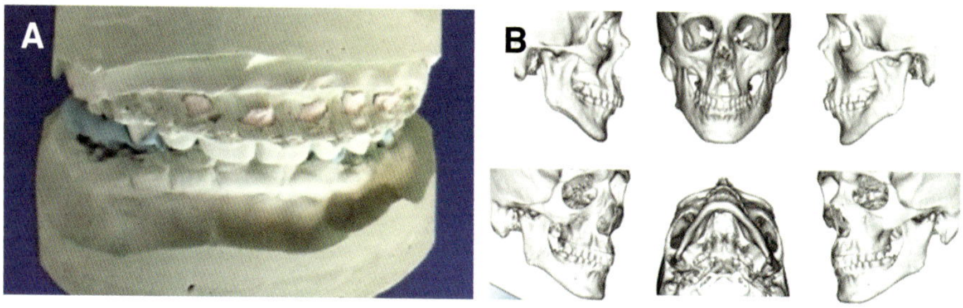

Fig. 1 (*A, B*): Dental casts with bite registration and CT scan are sent to the VSP company for MMA planning.

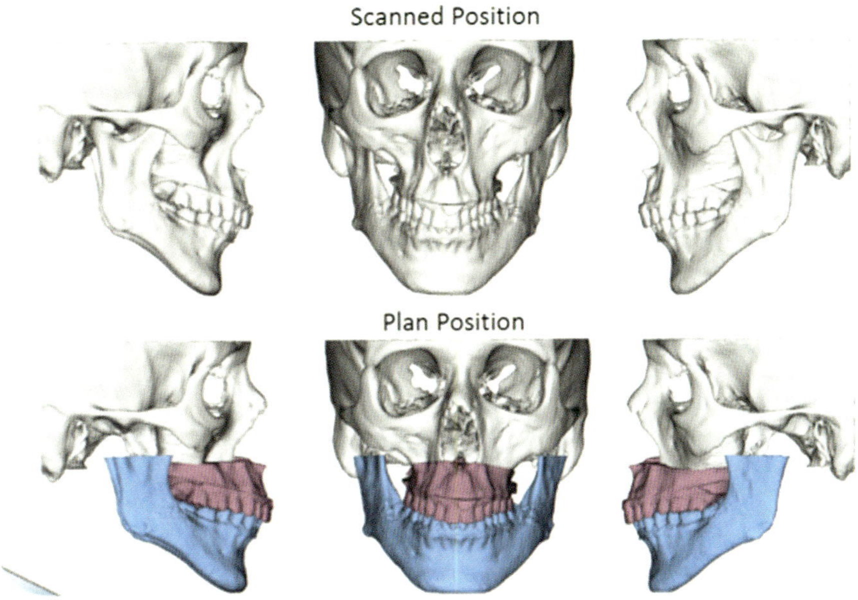

Fig. 2 Dental models are scanned and incorporated into the CT image. Virtual surgical workup competed with final positioning of the maxilla and mandible (maxilla and mandible have been advanced and rotated counterclockwise).

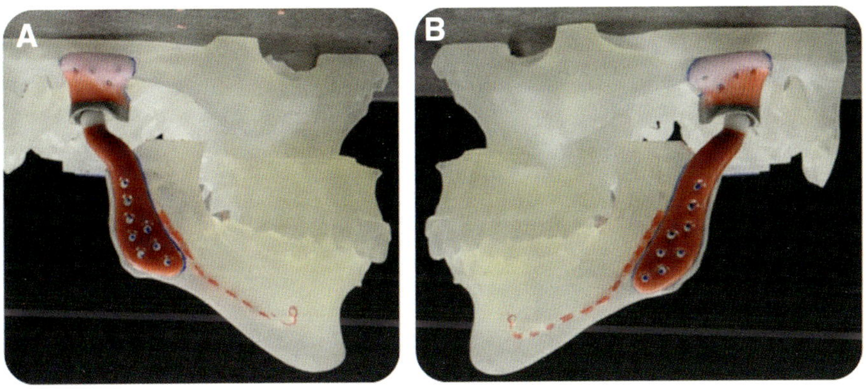

Fig. 3 (*A*, *B*) Right (*A*) and left (*B*) wax-up of the fossa and condyle by TMJ Concepts. (Ventura, CA)

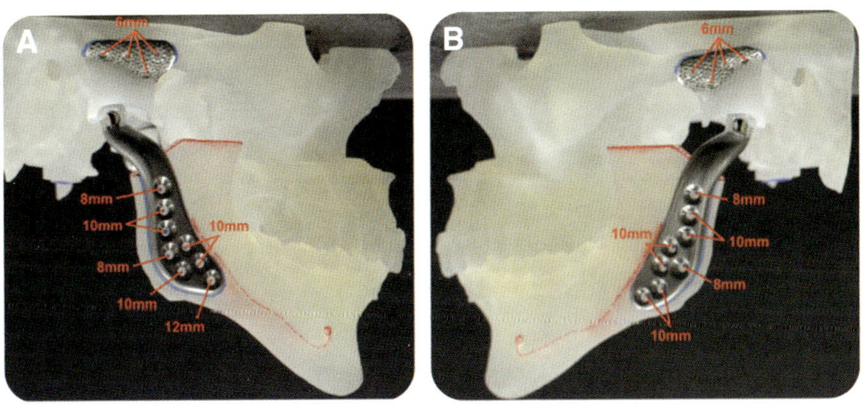

Fig. 4 (*A*, *B*) Fabricated right (*A*) and left (*B*) TMJs with the incorporated mandibular advancement.

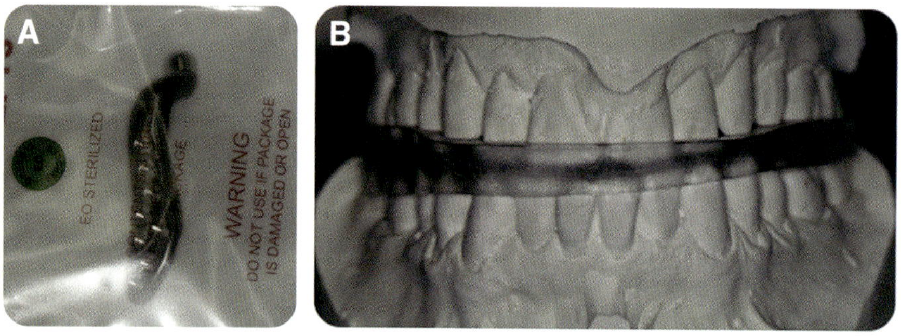

Fig. 5 (*A, B*) Stereolithic model and TMJ prosthesis and splints with dental models sent to the surgeon.

Surgical procedure

1. Bilateral TMJs are approached via a preauricular or endaural incision down through skin and subcutaneous tissue. A flap is raised above the supramuscular aponeurotic system (SMAS) and sutured anteriorly. The dissection continues just anterior to the tragal cartilage through the SMAS down to the level of the superficial layer of the temporalis fascia. A 2-cm incision is made through the temporalis fascia to expose the zygomatic arch and zygomatic root. Dissection is carried anteriorly along the arch to expose the eminence (Fig. 8).
2. An incision is made through the capsule down to the condyle. Condylar retractors are placed anteriorly and posteriorly to aid in visualization of the condylar neck. An osteotomy using BoneScalpel (Misonix, Farmingdale, NY, USA) is made through the condylar neck to minimize blood loss[18] (Fig. 9). The condylar head and articular disc are removed.
3. The submandibular incision is marked, and dissection is carried through skin, subcutaneous tissue, and superficial layer of the deep cervical fascia. The entire mandibular ramus is exposed up to the condylar neck, sigmoid notch, and coronoid. From the preauricular wound, an osteotomy is made 5 mm inferior to the sigmoid notch, across the coronoid and remaining condylar neck. The temporalis muscle is dissected off the coronoid process, and the bony complex is completely removed (Fig. 10).
4. The surgical steps outlined thus far are then carried out on the contralateral joint.
5. While maintaining a sterile field with additional towels, one member of the surgical team places the patient into intermaxillary fixation (IMF) using the intermediate occlusal splint. The contaminated towels are removed, and the mouth is again isolated with Tegaderm and 1010 drapes. The surgeon then rescrubs into the case.
6. Reconstruction is first focused on one of the TMJs, which includes insetting of the fossa and condylar prostheses, fat graft placement, and closure before starting on the contralateral side. This minimizes time of prosthetic exposure and possibility of infection.
7. The custom fossa prosthesis is placed and secured with 4 screws, after removal of bony interferences at the eminence

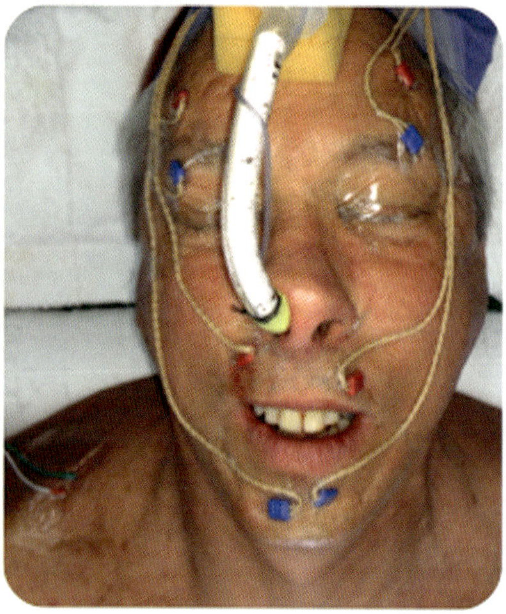

Fig. 6 Bilateral nerve integrity monitoring system (Medtronic, Minneapolis, MN) is placed to monitor the branches of the facial nerve.

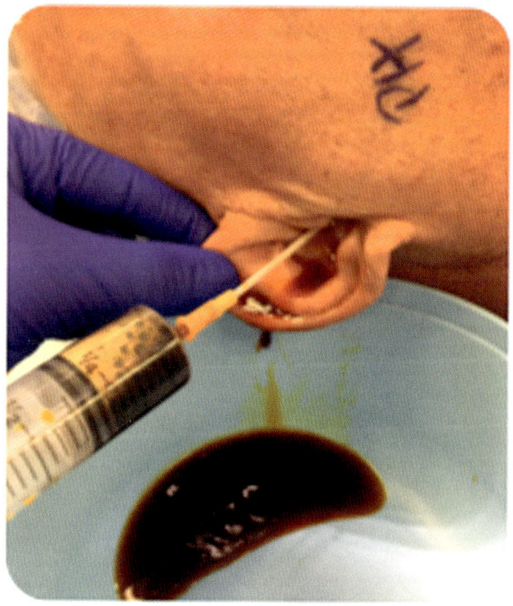

Fig. 7 The external auditory canal is irrigated with 300 ml of 1:1 ratio betadine and saline. The face and abdomen are then prepared with betadine and isolated with sterile towels and split sheet.

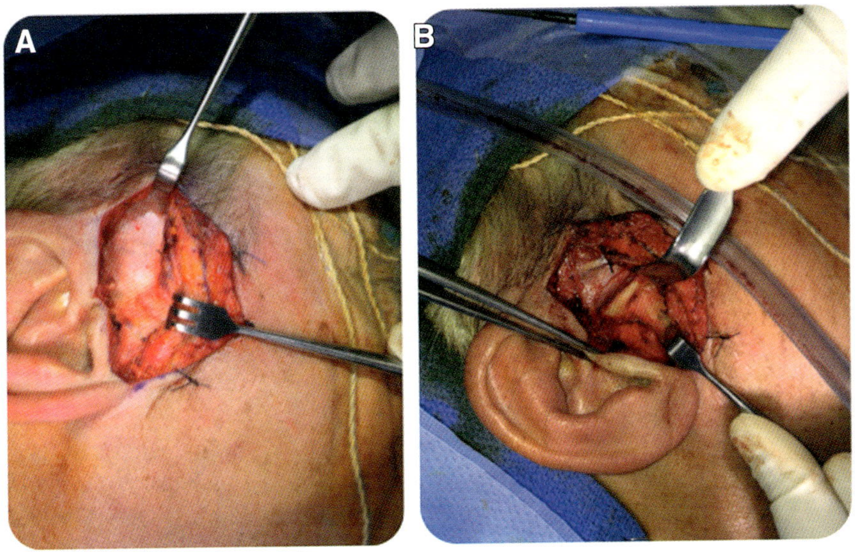

Fig. 8 (*A, B*) Dissection through the temporalis fascia to expose the zygomatic arch and eminence.

and fossa, if indicated on the stereolithic model. Next, the mandibular prosthesis is positioned so that it is flush on the ramus, and so that the condylar component is seated in the posterior aspect of the prosthetic fossa. The mandibular component is then secured with 6 screws (Fig. 11).

8. Fat graft is harvested from the abdomen at the lateral aspect, the umbilical area, or suprapubic region. A 2-cm incision is made through the skin and subcutaneous tissue, and fat is removed. The site is irrigated and closed after hemostasis is achieved.
9. The TMJ surgical site is irrigated; the fat graft is packed around the TMJ prosthesis (Fig. 12), and the incisions are closed in layers. The contralateral TMJ fossa and condylar prosthesis are next placed, packed with fat graft, and closed in a similar fashion.
10. The patient is released from IMF, and the intermediate splint is removed. Attention is directed to the maxillary surgery.
11. A K-wire is placed at level of nasion, and preoperative measurements with calipers are taken from K-wire to reproducible areas on the bilateral first molar, canine, and central incisors. Preoperative alar base is also measured.
12. A standard Le Fort I osteotomy is carried out. The incision is made through the maxillary vestibule from second premolar to contralateral premolar. A periosteal elevator is used to expose the anterior maxilla and lateral maxillary walls to the level of the pterygoid plates. The nasal mucosa is elevated from the piriform rim, lateral nasal wall, and nasal floor.
13. The maxillary osteotomy is cut from the buttress to the piriform rim. Interdental cuts are completed before downfracture of maxilla if multipiece maxillary osteotomy is indicated.
14. A double-guarded osteotome is used to separate the nasal septum from the nasal crest of the maxilla. A curved osteotome is used to divide the pterygoid-maxillary junction. A single guarded osteotome is used to cut through the lateral nasal wall.
15. The maxilla is downfractured and mobilized. Segmental osteotomies are then completed as indicated.
16. The final occlusal splint is inserted, and the maxilla is advanced to meet the newly positioned mandible and secured with IMF. The maxillomandibular complex is rotated counterclockwise, and bony interferences are

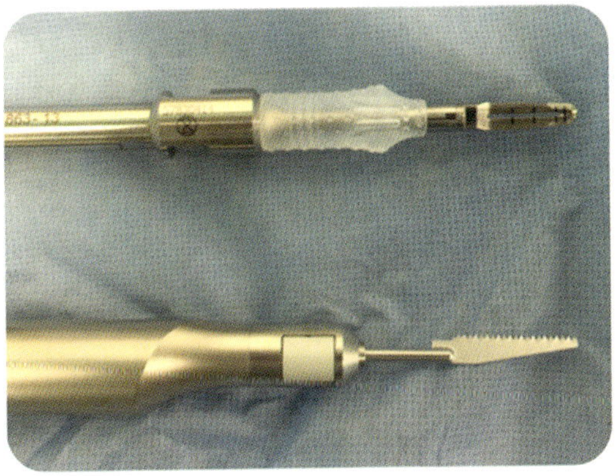

Fig. 9 BoneScalpel (top instrument; Misonix, Farmingdale, NY), piezoelectric device that preferentially cuts bone instead of soft tissue, is used to cut through the condylar neck to minimize blood loss.

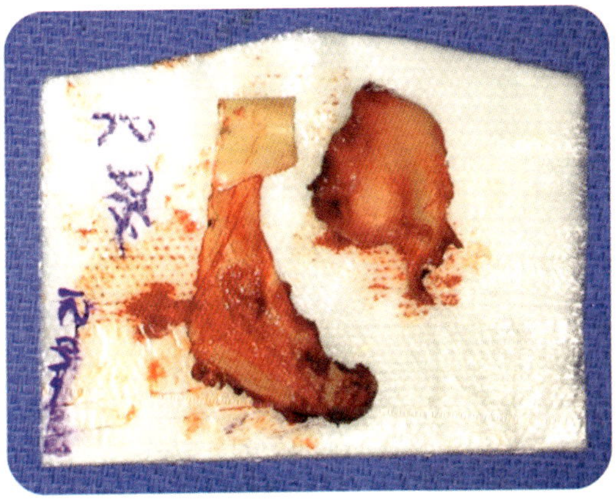

Fig. 10 Complete removal of the right condyle, coronoid process, and articular disc.

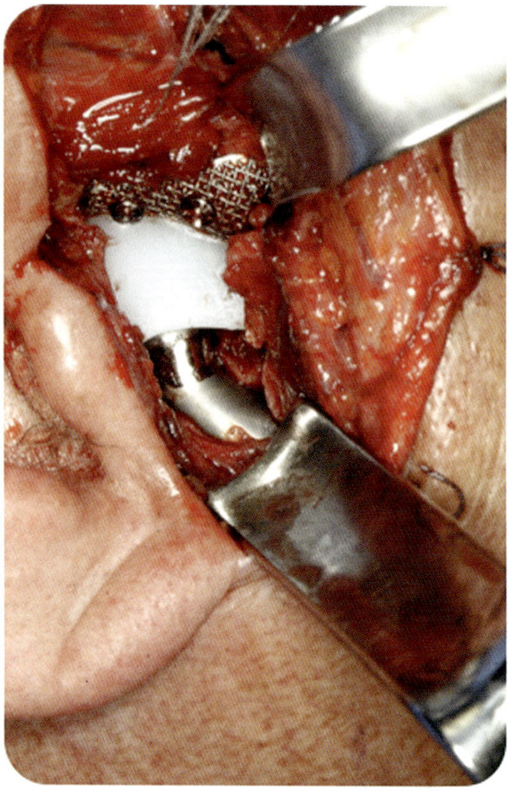

Fig. 11 Inset of the right fossa and condylar prosthesis.

removed to ensure adequate bony contact. Calipers are used to measure from the K-wire to the reproducible areas on the bilateral first molar, canine, and central incisors, and planned movements are confirmed, including elimination of a cant. The maxilla is rigidly fixated with 4 bone plates, one at the piriform region and one at the buttress bilaterally (Fig. 13). The alar base cinch suture is placed using 2-0 PDS suture and tightened to match the preoperative measurement. The maxillary incision is closed in a V-Y design to increase the upper lip length.

17. Additional procedures, such as genioplasty, turbinectomy, and lateral expansion pharyngoplasty, may be performed (Fig. 14).

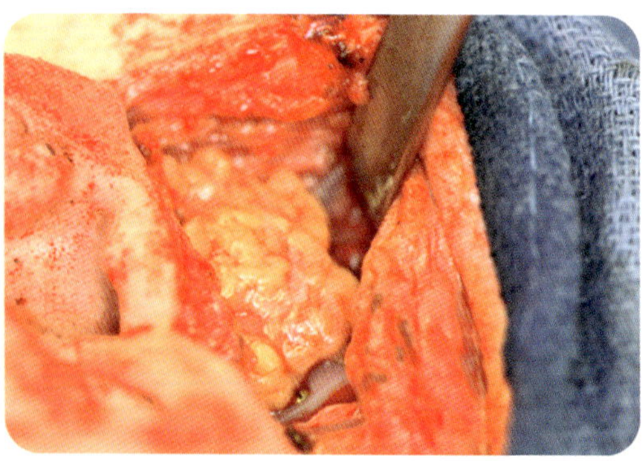

Fig. 12 Fat graft packed around the TMJ prosthesis. Good-quality abdominal fat is easy to procure and very beneficial for the prevention of heterotopic bone.

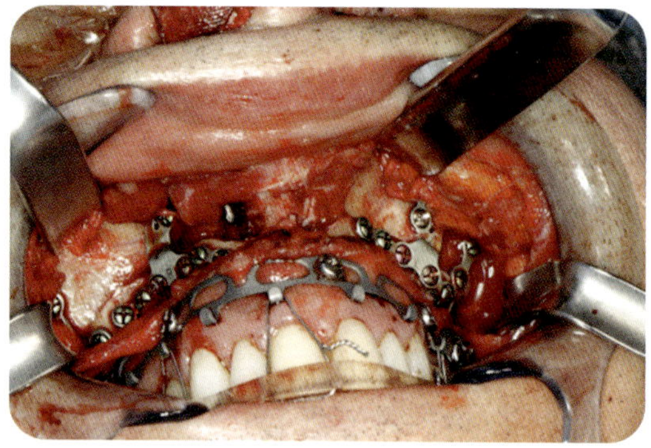

Fig. 13 Final splint has been placed and secured with IMF. The maxilla has been advanced, rotated counterclockwise, and rigidly fixated with plates and screws.

Potential complications

Undertaking TMJ reconstruction simultaneously with MMA for OSA is challenging and adds potential TMJ-specific complications to the surgical risk. The complications and treatment of the Le Fort I osteotomy are well documented.[19,20] This section discusses TMJ-specific complications.

1. Prosthetic joint dislocation: Prosthetic joint dislocation risk is highest in the first 48 hours (Fig. 15). Maintenance of IMF for up to 2 weeks is advised. Displacement is treated by manually manipulation.
2. Periprosthetic joint infection (PJI): The diagnosis of PJI is challenging due to limitations in imaging and negative laboratory findings. Acute TMJ infections can be managed with IV antibiotics and surgical debridement.[21] Chronic PJI is treated with a PICC (peripherally inserted central catheter) line and antibiotics for 4 to 6 weeks, removal of the prosthesis, and placement of an antibiotic-impregnated acrylic spacer (stage I surgery), followed by reconstruction with a new prosthesis after 3 months (stage II surgery).
3. Hardware failure: Each fossa component should have 4 screws, and each mandibular component should have at least 6 screws. If hardware failure is suspected, a new custom prosthesis must be designed to replace the old hardware.
4. Hardware design error: Patients with teeth worn flat and with large centric relation-centric occlusion shifts are vulnerable to not capturing centric occlusion during CT scan. Always send stone models of the upper and lower

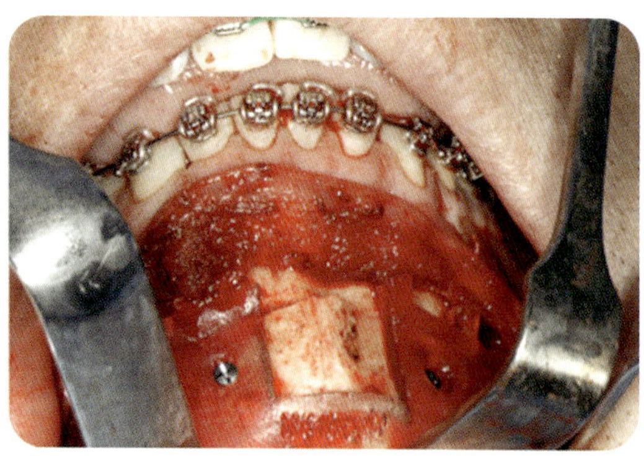

Fig. 14 Adjuvant procedures such as genioglossus advancement may be performed if indicated.

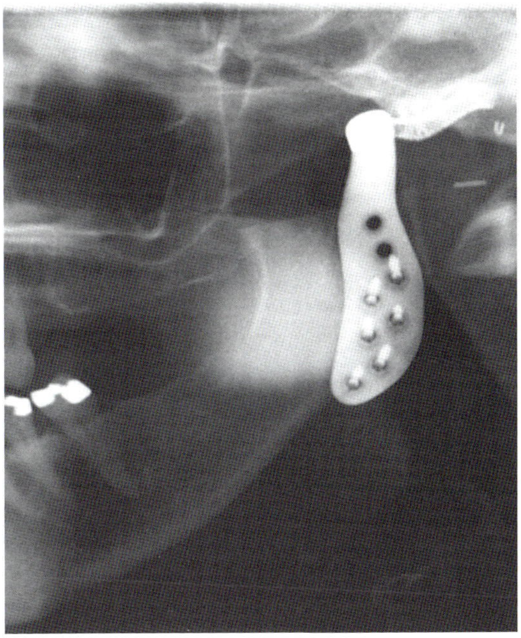

Fig. 15 The mandibular component of the TMJ Concepts (Ventura, CA) custom prosthesis is dislocated anterior to the prosthetic fossa on postoperative day 2.

arches and a bite registration to TMJ Concepts for digital incorporation into the CT scan (Fig. 16).

5. Metal allergy: It is estimated that 10% to 15% of the general population has a metal allergy.[22] Query patients about possible metal allergies and refer to an allergist if necessary.
6. Heterotopic bone formation: Scar tissue and reactive bone formation can occur around the articulating areas of the prosthesis. The use of autogenous fat packed around the head of the prosthesis has significantly decreased the risk of heterotopic bone formation (see Fig. 12).
7. Malocclusion: Posterior and anterior open bites may result from either an error in positioning the mandibular component of the prosthesis or improper placement and stability of the maxillary surgery (Fig. 17). Manage postoperative malocclusion with guiding elastics initially for up to 4 to 6 weeks and possible orthodontic therapy. Repositioning of the maxilla and/or the mandibular components of the prosthesis may be required.
8. Bleeding: Most arterial bleeding arises from the middle meningeal and posterior deep temporal arteries, branches of the internal maxillary artery, or direct injury to the maxillary artery. Use of a piezoelectric or ultrasonic bone saw can significantly reduce total blood loss[18] (see Fig. 9). Management of uncontrolled arterial bleeding from the internal maxillary artery may require dissection down to the external carotid artery and subsequent ligation.

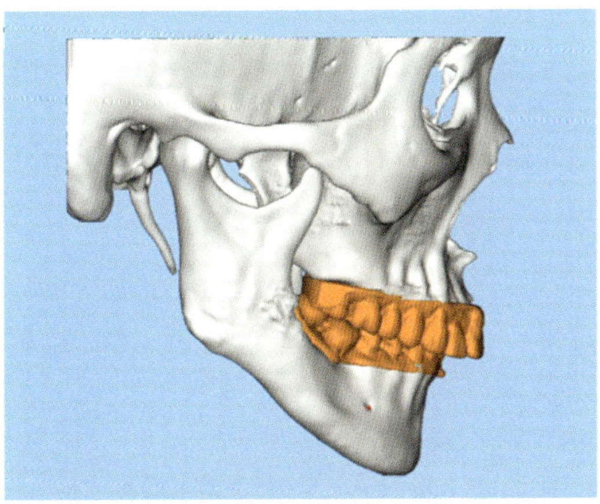

Fig. 16 Stone model integration into the CT scan. For patients who have severe dental attrition or who have a large centric occlusion - centric relation (CO-CR) slide, a surgical splint made through computer-aided design and computer-aided manufacturing (CAD/CAM) methods is strongly advised, even when the plan is to maintain the patient's existing occlusion MMA with bilateral total joint replacement.

Pearls and pitfalls

1. Ensure the orthodontic brackets, wires, and hooks are secure and can withstand the intraoperative force demands. If the hooks loosen or the brackets disengage intraoperatively, remove the orthodontic appliances and place either a traditional or bone-supported hybrid IMF.
2. Counterclockwise rotation of the maxillomandibular complex provides larger increases in airway dimension and minimizes the negative esthetic effects of a large, straight anterior movement. It is critical to not overdo the counterclockwise rotation because the bilateral TMJ complexes will not be able to rotate enough to close the occlusion, leading to apertognathia.
3. Inform patient of the potential need for preorthodontic and postorthodontic treatment.
4. Proper sequencing of the bilateral TMJ reconstructions allows for decreased swelling and risk of infection. The surgical team should perform bilateral hard tissue resections first, followed by placing the prosthetic joint on one side

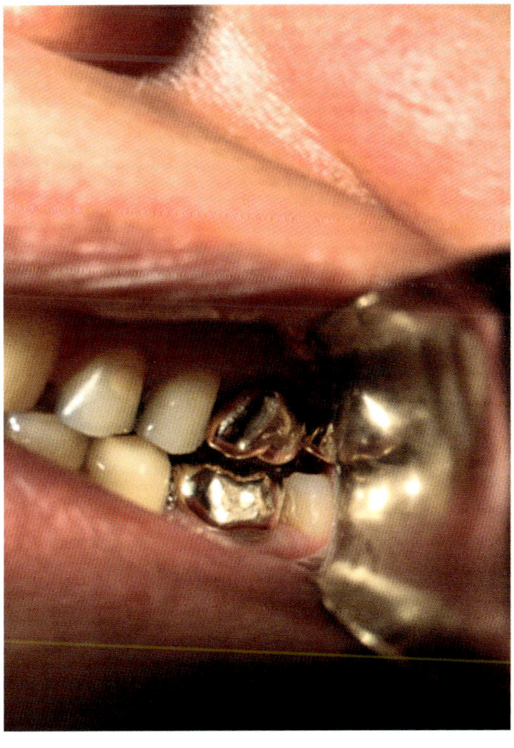

Fig. 17 A 1-mm ipsilateral posterior open bite is noted on postoperative day 1, after placing a total joint prosthesis.

and closing the wound. Next, the prosthetic joint is placed on the other side, and the wound is closed.

5. Wash out the ear with povidone-iodine solution (see Fig. 7), place gauze impregnated with petroleum jelly into the external auditory meatus, and suture the tragus closed (Fig. 18) to minimize contamination originating from the external auditory meatus.
6. The condylar prosthesis has a medially directed curve as it transitions from the ramus up toward the fossa. To prevent a gap formation between the prosthesis and the osteotimized mandibular bone (Fig. 19), place one screw on the inferior aspect of the prosthesis, leave it loose, and then place one as superiorly as possible. This helps in adapting the prosthesis to the lateral surface of the mandible. In addition, ensure that sufficient ramus bone reduction occurs to allow for clearance of the medial curve to ensure appropriate adaptation of the prosthesis.

Immediate postoperative care

1. Place a thin coat of antibiotic ointment and a nonstick dressing over skin incisions. Cover mandibular incisions with gauze dressing and Tegaderm.
2. Wrap a firm compression bandage around the head for 1 to 2 days to minimize risk of hematoma formation.
3. Minimize swelling with perioperative steroids and ice packs.
4. Patient should be in heavy elastic traction to prevent TMJ dislocation.
5. Maintain IMF for 1 to 2 weeks postoperatively for comfort and to prevent shift in occlusion due to surgical edema around the prosthetic joints.
6. The final occlusal splint is kept in place for up to 4 weeks and occlusion is managed with guiding elastics.
7. The antibiotic selected should cover skin, ear, and oral flora. An antibiotic regimen consisting of IV (hospital course) and oral (after discharge) for a total of 7 days is recommended, although there is no strong evidence for this practice.

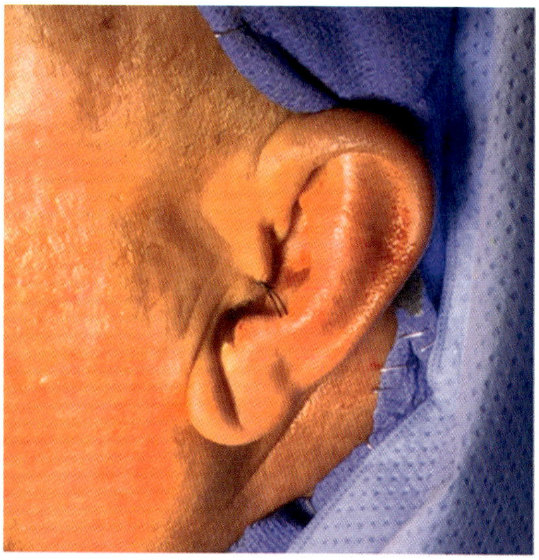

Fig. 18 The tragus is closed with a single suture to prevent gauze impregnated with petroleum jelly packing from falling into the wound and potentially contaminating the surgical field.

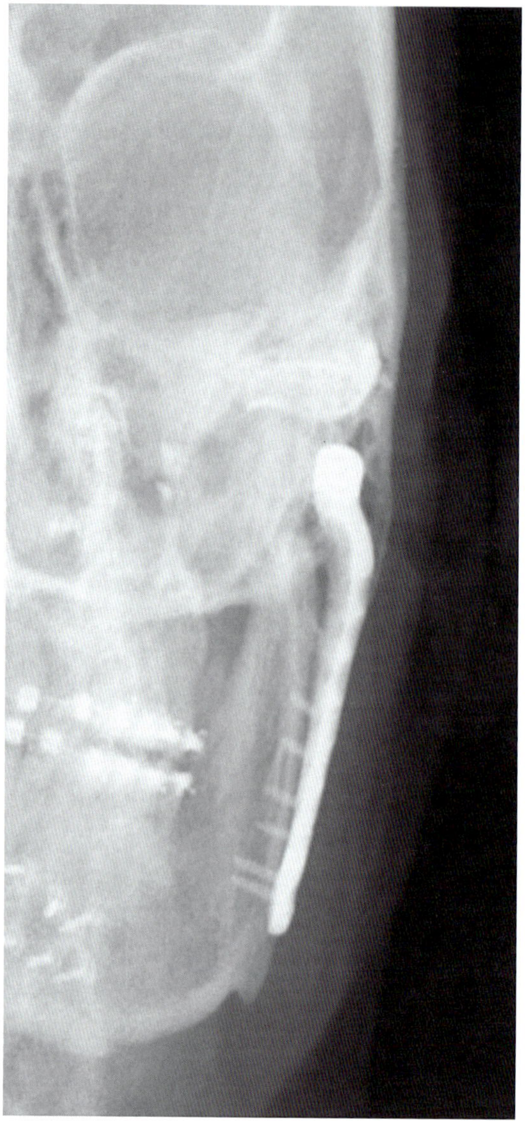

Fig. 19 The prosthesis is slightly lifted off the ramus of the mandible in this PA view.

8. Postoperative radiographs are done before hospital discharge and include panoramic, lateral, and posteroanterior (PA) cephalometric radiographs.
9. Educate regarding hand hygiene, incision care, shaving, showering, and hair washing. Incisions should not be handled by the patient except to apply a thin layer of an antibiotic ointment.
10. A liquid diet is required until the IMF is released and the splint is removed. Slow advancement of the diet is advised.

Rehabilitation and recovery

1. Physical therapy should begin within 4 weeks postoperatively. This allows for the surgical swelling and pain to subside, but is timed before scar tissue forms and muscle spasm begins. The therapist needs to be made aware that the stability of the maxilla is not set at this early stage. Specific duration of physical therapy treatment has not been defined; however, 12 treatment sessions should be the minimum.

2. Occlusal stability is a crucial element to maintain surgical stability. Postsurgical orthodontics is often necessary to balance out the occlusion.
3. Muscle spasms and pain can be treated with either onabotulinumtoxinA or incobotulinumtoxinA injections administered at 6 to 8 weeks postoperatively. Standard TMD botulinumtoxin treatment consists of 3 injection points to the inferior border of the masseter muscle and 2 injection points to the anterior superior aspect of the temporalis muscle, 10 units each location for a total of 100 units.
4. Self-directed jaw opening exercises can be more aggressively performed as maxillary osteotomy reaches full stability. There are several devices on the market designed for jaw-opening exercises, which should be performed a minimum of 3 sessions per day with a goal maximal incisal opening (MIO) of at least 35 mm.

Clinical results in the literature

TMD and OSA are distinct pathologic entities with direct anatomic associations resulting in synergistically worsening symptoms, but the underlying mechanisms remain poorly understood. One explanation of the association between TMD and OSA can be seen in patients with idiopathic condylar resorption leading to airway obstruction resulting from collapsed posterior mandibular height and clockwise rotation. By correcting the posterior mandibular height through either distraction osteogenesis or TJR, the mandible is rotated counterclockwise alleviating the airway obstruction.[23,24] However, there is a paucity of literature looking at sleep studies and sleep and TMJ symptom changes in patients who have undergone bilateral TJR with MMA surgery.

TMJ and OSA evaluation requires a multimodality diagnostic approach to determine ideal surgical intervention. DISE is a dynamic evaluation of the airway at 4 different levels,[17] which guides the clinician's decision making in tailoring the surgical treatment options.[15] DISE is an integral aspect of OSA diagnosis that should be used to further ensure the appropriateness in selecting bilateral TJR and MMA as the treatment option, and further research is needed in this area.

MMA for the treatment of OSA has been well studied and documented over the years.[25–28] TMJs are the foundation for stability and long-term success of MMA surgery. Pathologic TMJs can lead to unsatisfactory MMA results and relapse. Thus, TMJ pathologic condition should be considered if a patient presents with high occlusal plane angle, progressive anterior open bites, changes in jaw relationship, and myofascial or TMJ pain. Over the past 40 years, major advancements have been made in TMJ surgery that have reduced operative complications, decreased the morbidity, and increased postoperative success. Such advances in TMJ surgery include custom fabricated joint prostheses, harvesting and placement of fat graft at the joint to prevent heterotopic bone formation,[29] minimizing prosthesis exposure during insetting to reduce risk of infection, and use of ultrasonic hand piece to reduce bleeding.[18] TMJ reconstruction creates rigid struts that maintain vertical dimension allowing predictable results to treat pathologic and painful TMJs and improve MIO, jaw function, and quality of life.[10,30–33]

Few studies have shown the degree of changes in the airway space following bilateral TMJ reconstruction with concomitant MMA. However, these studies did not evaluate for the effect of the surgical procedure on the sleep symptoms and PSG results. Coleta and colleagues[12] demonstrated long-term stability of the bilateral TMJ reconstruction and immediate increase in oropharyngeal airway dimension with menton advancing an average of 18.4 mm. Gonçalves[13] and colleagues showed 3-dimensional airway space changes and long-term stability following TJR and MMA in 30 female patients. The average change in airway surface area was 179.5 mm^2 and volume was 6302.6 mm^3. Further research is needed to elucidate the effect of the bilateral TMJ reconstruction with concomitant MMA on the sleep symptoms and PSG results.

Summary

The various diagnostic modalities, such as clinical examination, imaging, and DISE, should be used together to provide a comprehensive airway and TMJ evaluation to select appropriate surgical treatment option. VSP is an accurate method to optimize MMA movements in setting of TMJ reconstruction. Patients with TMD and OSA who are intolerant of medical therapies can be treated effectively with custom TMJ reconstruction in combination with MMA.

References

1. Wolk R, Somers VK. Sleep and the metabolic syndrome. Exp Physiol 2007;92(1):67–78.
2. Einhorn D, Stewart DA, Erman MK, et al. Prevalence of sleep apnea in a population of adults with type 2 diabetes mellitus. Endocr Pract 2007;13(4):355–62.
3. Dubrovsky B, Raphael KG, Lavigne GJ, et al. Polysomnographic investigation of sleep and respiratory parameters in women with temporomandibular pain disorders. J Clin Sleep Med 2014;10(2):195 201.
4. Tay DKL, Pang KP. Clinical phenotype of South-East Asian temporomandibular disorder patients with upper airway resistance syndrome. J Oral Rehabil 2018;45(1):25–33.
5. Sanders AE, Essick GK, Fillingim R, et al. Sleep apnea symptoms and risk of temporomandibular disorder: OPPERA cohort. J Dent Res 2013;92(7 Suppl):70S–7S.
6. Schendel SA, Powell NB. Surgical orthognathic management of sleep apnea. J Craniofac Surg 2007;18(4):902–11.
7. Caples SM, Rowley JA, Prinsell JR, et al. Surgical modifications of the upper airway for obstructive sleep apnea in adults: a systematic review and meta-analysis. Sleep 2010;33(10):1396–407.
8. Mercuri LG, Wolford LM, Sanders B, et al. Long-term follow-up of the CAD/CAM patient fitted total temporomandibular joint reconstruction system. J Oral Maxillofac Surg 2002;60(12):1440–8.
9. Wolford LM. Computer-assisted surgical simulation for concomitant temporomandibular joint custom-fitted total joint reconstruction and orthognathic surgery. Atlas Oral Maxillofac Surg Clin North Am 2016;24(1):55–66.
10. Wolford LM, Mercuri LG, Schneiderman ED, et al. Twenty-year follow-up study on a patient-fitted temporomandibular joint prosthesis: the Techmedica/TMJ Concepts device. J Oral Maxillofac Surg 2015;73(5):952–60.
11. Wolford LM, Pinto LP, Cárdenas LE, et al. Outcomes of treatment with custom-made temporomandibular joint total joint prostheses and maxillomandibular counter-clockwise rotation. Proc (Bayl Univ Med Cent) 2008;21(1):18–24.
12. Coleta KE, Wolford LM, Gonçalves JR, et al. Maxillo-mandibular counter-clockwise rotation and mandibular advancement with TMJ Concepts total joint prostheses: part II—airway changes and stability. Int J Oral Maxillofac Surg 2009;38(3):228–35.
13. Gonçalves JR, Gomes LC, Vianna AP, et al. Airway space changes after maxillomandibular counterclockwise rotation and mandibular advancement with TMJ Concepts® total joint prostheses: three-dimensional assessment. Int J Oral Maxillofac Surg 2013;42(8):1014–22.

14. Schendel SA, Jacobson R, Khalessi S. Airway growth and development: a computerized 3-dimensional analysis. J Oral Maxillofac Surg 2012;70(9):2174–83.
15. Lechner M, Wilkins D, Kotecha B. A review on drug-induced sedation endoscopy - technique, grading systems and controversies. Sleep Med Rev 2018;41:141–8.
16. Yegïn Y, Çelik M, Kaya KH, et al. Comparison of drug-induced sleep endoscopy and Müller's maneuver in diagnosing obstructive sleep apnea using the VOTE classification system. Braz J Otorhinolaryngol 2017;83(4):445–50.
17. Kezirian EJ, Hohenhorst W, de Vries N. Drug-induced sleep endoscopy: the VOTE classification. Eur Arch Otorhinolaryngol 2011;268(8):1233–6.
18. Silva R, Gupta R, Tartaglia G, et al. Benefits of using the ultrasonic BoneScalpel™ in temporomandibular joint reconstruction. J Craniomaxillofac Surg 2017;45(3):401–7.
19. Garg S, Kaur S. Evaluation of post-operative complication rate of le fort i osteotomy: a retrospective and prospective study. J Maxillofac Oral Surg 2014;13(2):120–7.
20. Olate S, Sigua E, Asprino L, et al. Complications in orthognathic surgery. J Craniofac Surg 2018;29(2):e158–61.
21. Wolford LM, Rodrigues DB, McPhillips A. Management of the infected temporomandibular joint total joint prosthesis. J Oral Maxillofac Surg 2010;68(11):2810–23.
22. Schram SE, Warshaw EM, Laumann A. Nickel hypersensitivity: a clinical review and call to action. Int J Dermatol 2010;49(2):115–25.
23. Wolford LM. Idiopathic condylar resorption of the temporomandibular joint in teenage girls (cheerleaders syndrome). Proc (Bayl Univ Med Cent) 2001;14(3):246–52.
24. Yuen H, Rossouw PE, Wolford LM, et al. Pharyngeal airway space changes after condylar replacement and mandibular advancement surgery. J Oral Maxillofac Surg 2018;76(6):1165–74.
25. Li KK, Powell NB, Riley RW, et al. Long-term results of maxillomandibular advancement surgery. Sleep Breath 2000;4(3):137–40.
26. Camacho M, Liu SY, Certal V, et al. Large maxillomandibular advancements for obstructive sleep apnea: an operative technique evolved over 30 years. J Craniomaxillofac Surg 2015;43(7):1113–8.
27. Holty JE, Guilleminault C. Maxillomandibular advancement for the treatment of obstructive sleep apnea: a systematic review and meta-analysis. Sleep Med Rev 2010;14(5):287–97.
28. Liu SY, Huon LK, Iwasaki T, et al. Efficacy of maxillomandibular advancement examined with drug-induced sleep endoscopy and computational fluid dynamics airflow modeling. Otolaryngol Head Neck Surg 2016;154(1):189–95.
29. Wolford LM, Karras SC. Autologous fat transplantation around temporomandibular joint total joint prostheses: preliminary treatment outcomes. J Oral Maxillofac Surg 1997;55(3):245–51 [discussion: 251–2].
30. Mercuri LG, Edibam NR, Giobbie-Hurder A. Fourteen-year follow-up of a patient-fitted total temporomandibular joint reconstruction system. J Oral Maxillofac Surg 2007;65(6):1140–8.
31. Mercuri LG, Ali FA, Woolson R. Outcomes of total alloplastic replacement with periarticular autogenous fat grafting for management of reankylosis of the temporomandibular joint. J Oral Maxillofac Surg 2008;66(9):1794–803.
32. Mercuri LG. Subjective and objective outcomes in patients reconstructed with a custom-fitted alloplastic temporomandibular joint prosthesis. J Oral Maxillofac Surg 1999;57(12):1427–30.
33. Dela Coleta KE, Wolford LM, Gonçalves JR, et al. Maxillomandibular counter-clockwise rotation and mandibular advancement with TMJ Concepts total joint prostheses: part I—skeletal and dental stability. Int J Oral Maxillofac Surg 2009;38(2):126–38.

Upper Airway (Hypoglossal Nerve) Stimulation for Treatment of Obstructive Sleep Apnea

Rishi Jay Gupta, DDS, MD, MBA [a,b,c], Deepak Kademani, DMD, MD [d], Stanley Yung-Chuan Liu, DDS, MD [e,*]

KEYWORDS

• Obstructive sleep apnea • Upper airway stimulation • Hypoglossal nerve stimulation • Sleep surgery
• Drug induced sleep endoscopy • Implant

KEY POINTS

- Obstructive sleep apnea is a multilevel process consisting of physiologic and anatomic obstructive patterns leading to partial or complete collapse of the upper airway and resulting comorbidities.
- Studies have shown apnea-hypopnea index (AHI) response rate of 75% (AHI less than 20 events per hour and overall >50% reduction) and improvement in quality of life in patients treated with upper airway stimulation (UAS).
- UAS is indicated in patients with positive airway pressure failure, who are 22 years of age or older, with AHI 15 to 65, with body mass index less than or equal to 32 and anatomy amenable to implantation and likelihood of high success.
- Drug-induced sleep endoscopy is an essential evaluation step to exclude patients with retropalatal concentric collapse.
- Preparation of cranial nerve XII and determination of functional breakpoint to exclude the lateral XII branches and include the medial XII branches are critical to optimize surgical success.

Introduction

OSA is characterized by repeated partial or complete collapse of the upper airway during sleep.[1] Cessation of breathing leads to nocturnal hypoxemia and arousals resulting in increase in mortality[2] and comorbidities, such as hypertension, stroke, myocardial infarction, and diabetes.[3,4] OSA has emerged as a serious medical condition with considerable health and social ramifications. Positive airway pressure (PAP) is the first-line medical management of OSA with high efficacy of successful treatment. Compliance with PAP therapy remains low, however, approximately 50% to 60%, resulting in many untreated patients with OSA. Patients with OSA who are intolerant of PAP can be treated by other interventions, such as oral appliance therapy and upper airway surgical options.[5,6]

A detailed perioperative assessment of patients with OSA, including clinical examination, drug-induced sleep endoscopy (DISE), and radiographic analysis, is critical to ensure selection of the most effective surgical treatment option depending on the level of airway obstruction. Patients with multilevel obstruction may be treated with traditional Stanford protocol phase 1, consisting of nasal, palatal, and tongue base surgery; maxillomandibular advancement (MMA); or upper airway stimulation (UAS). The treatment selection depends on the severity of OSA and likelihood of surgical success.

Upper airway therapy through the neuromuscular stimulation of the hypoglossal nerve and genioglossus muscle has emerged as an effective treatment option and must be included in the surgeon's armamentarium for treatment of OSA.[7–10] This therapy utilizes an implantable device with a stimulation electrode placed around the protrusive branches of the hypoglossal nerve and a sensor lead placed in the intercostal space to detect inspiration. The patient-specific programmable device stimulates the hypoglossal nerve during timed inspiration to alleviate the airway obstruction in patients with moderate or severe OSA.

UAS has been shown to affect the retroglossal and retropalatal areas be increasing the airway in an anterior-posterior direction.[11,12] By stimulating the hypoglossal nerve, the tongue base protrudes due to genioglossus muscle activation, resulting in opening of the airway in the retroglossal region. The exact mechanism of the effects on the retropalatal areas is not entirely known; however, a concentric palatal collapse is a contraindication to UAS therapy.[11,13,14] Various UAS devices have been developed over the

Disclosure Statement: The authors have nothing to disclose.

[a] Oral and Maxillofacial Surgery Section, Department of Dental Service, San Francisco VA Health Care System, 4150 Clement Street (160), San Francisco, CA 94121, USA
[b] Department of Oral and Maxillofacial Surgery, University of California, San Francisco, 707 Parnassus Ave, San Francisco, CA 94143, USA
[c] Department of Otolaryngology Head and Neck Surgery, University of California, Davis, 2521 Stockton Blvd, Sacramento, CA 95817, USA
[d] Head and Neck Oncologic and Reconstructive Surgery, Department of Oral and Maxillofacial Surgery, North Memorial Medical Center, Minneapolis, MN 55422, USA
[e] Division of Sleep Surgery, Department of Otolaryngology, Stanford Sleep Surgery Fellowship, Stanford University School of Medicine, 801 Welch Road, Stanford, CA 94305, USA
* Corresponding author.
E-mail address: ycliu@stanford.edu

Atlas Oral Maxillofacial Surg Clin N Am 27 (2019) 53–58
1061-3315/19/Published by Elsevier Inc.
https://doi.org/10.1016/j.cxom.2018.11.004

years, with the technology subsequently modified.[15] Most recently, Inspire Medical Systems (Maple Grove, Minnesota) has obtained Food and Drug Administration approval for a UAS device, and a 5-year Stimulation Therapy for Apnea Reduction (STAR) outcome study showed improvement in sleepiness (Epworth Sleepiness Scale [ESS]) and quality of life (Functional Outcomes of Sleep Questionnaire [FOSQ]), with normalization of scores increasing from 33% to 78% and 15% to 67%, respectively, and showed an apnea-hypopnea index (AHI) response rate of 75% (AHI <20 events per hour and overall >50% reduction).[16]

Surgeons need to have thorough understanding of the preoperative and surgical protocols to optimize postoperative outcomes. This article describes the steps required for preoperative assessment, diagnostic work-up, performance of implantation of the UAS device, and postoperative management.

Surgical technique

Diagnostic work-up

A baseline polysomnography (PSG) or home sleep study is obtained to first diagnose the severity of OSA. After confirmation of OSA, comprehensive clinical, radiographic, and endoscopic diagnostic work-up is performed to determine the appropriate selection of sleep surgical options. The clinical examination consists of evaluation of the nasal passages, oropharyngeal space, and retroglossal area. DISE is performed to characterize airway collapse pattern. The pattern and degree of collapse is scored according to the velum, oropharyngeal, tongue base, and epiglottis classification.[14,17]

UAS indications:

1. PAP failure
2. 22 years of age or older
3. AHI 15 to 65
4. Body mass index (BMI) ≤32
5. Anatomy amenable to implantation and likelihood of high success

UAS contraindications:

1. Sleep study showing greater than 25% central or mixed apneas
2. Concentric palatal collapse seen on DISE[11,13,14]
3. Unable to operate the therapy
4. Pregnancy
5. Preexisting anatomic alterations or neurologic disorders
6. Patients who require MRI
   a. Inspire Model 3024: MRI is contraindicated because it may cause tissue damage and/or damage to the UAS device.
   b. Inspire Model 3028: if certain conditions are met, patients may undergo an MRI scan on head and extremities.

UAS precautions:

1. BMI greater than 32 may be associated with decreased likelihood of surgical success.
2. Diathermy (primarily used in physical therapy): do not use shortwave diathermy, microwave diathermy, or therapeutic ultrasound diathermy on patients with a neurostimulation system.
3. Electromagnetic compatibility and interference, electrocautery, irradiation, lithotripsy, radiofrequency ablation, radiograph, fluoroscopy, ultrasonics, defibrillation, or radition can adversely affect the UAS system.

Preparation and patient positioning

1. The patient is taken to the operating room and is placed in the supine position, and short-acting muscle relaxers are used prior to intubating orally or nasally.
2. Patient is given dexamethasone and preoperative antibiotics, such as IV cefazolin, within 60 minutes of first incision.
3. Nerve Monitoring System (NIM) (Medtronic, Minneapolis, Minnesota) monitors the tongue response by utilizing sensor leads (Xomed 82273049) and bipolar simulating probe (Xomed 8225401).
   a. Inclusion: NIM blue electrode is placed using a Debakey forceps right of the midline and in the floor of the mouth by plunging into the genioglossus muscle (avoid frenulum and salivary duct). This ensures inclusion of the protrusive muscles (genioglossus oblique [GGo] and genioglossus horizontal [GGh]) and of the tongue narrowing/flattening muscles (transverse and vertical [T/V]), which are innervated by the medial branches of XII.
   b. Exclusion: NIM red electrode is placed using a Debakey 5 cm from the tip of the tongue and inserted into the ventrolateral and submucosal surface of the tongue. This ensures exclusion of the retractor muscles (styloglossus [SG] and hyoglossus [HG]), which are innervated by the lateral branches of XII.
4. Bite block is placed to hold the mouth open to visualize the tongue during device testing at the end of the case.
5. Shoulder roll and jelly donut used to extend the head to the left for optimal surgical access. Keep the arm on the implant side free of IV, pulse oximetry, and blood pressure cuff and loosely tuck.
6. The 3 surgical sites are then marked at the stimulation lead incision (neck), implantable pulse generator (IPG) pocket incision (superior chest), and sense lead incision (inferolateral chest).
   a. Stimulation lead incision: 4-cm to 6-cm incision is marked midway along the length of the right mandible and midway between the hyoid and mandible while staying 1 cm from the midline.
   b. IPG pocket incision: 5.5-cm incision is marked 5 cm inferior to clavicle and midway between the sternum and deltopectoral groove.
   c. Sense lead incision: palpate the 5th (±1) rib using inferolateral margin of pectoralis major as a landmark; 4-cm to 6-cm incision marked following the curvature of the rib approximately 5 cm lateral from a line straight down from the nipple.
7. The face, neck, and chest are then prepped with betadine. Sterile towels are secured with staples to isolate surgical sites. Adhesive drape (Ioban [3M, St. Paul, Minnesota]) is placed over exposed skin to maintain aseptic technique at all 3 surgical sites. A transparent drape (1012 [3M]) is then placed across the Ioban to cover the oral cavity while ensuring visual access to the tongue. A split sheet is then secured over the drapes.

Surgical procedure

1. Neck incision is carried through the skin, platysma, and superficial layer of the deep cervical fascia while avoiding the marginal mandibular branch of the facial nerve. The

submandibular gland is located, carefully dissected at the inferior and anterior aspect away from the mylohyoid muscle, and retracted posteriorly.

2. Identify the anterior belly of digastric muscles and trace back to the digastric tendon. Tunnel under the digastric tendon toward the mylohyoid muscle to provide a path for the stimulating lead. Place a vessel loop around the digastric tendon and retract inferiorly. Free the posterior margin of the mylohyoid muscle and retract the muscle anteriorly.
3. By retracting the submandibular gland posteriorly, the mylohyoid muscle anteriorly, and the digastric tendon inferiorly, the hypoglossal nerve (cranial nerve [CN] XII) can be visualized, which lies superficial to the HG muscle and deep to the mylohyoid muscle. Surgeons must be careful not to injure important structures in the field, such as the lingual nerve and submandibular duct. Once the hypoglossal nerve is identified, the ranine vein may need to be ligated and divided because it often lies over the nerve.
4. Identify the hypoglossal nerve (CN XII) and the functional breakpoint using stimulation and NIM monitoring. The goal is to separate the branches of XII that produce a uniform protrusive and stiffened tongue motion from the branches of XII that cause tongue retraction. Surgeons should work counterclockwise along the hypoglossal nerve from inferior to posterior (geniohyoid [GH], GGh, GGo, T/V, HG, and SG) and stimulate the individual branches within the main trunk to exclude the lateral XII branches (HG and SG) and include the medial XII branches (GGh, GGo, and T/V) and, when possible, the C1 branch from XII to the GH muscle (Fig. 1).
5. Use a fine vessel loop to isolate the inclusion branches of XII and validate with NIM. It is important to minimize dissection on the nerve to prevent neuropraxia. While placing gentle traction on the nerve, the surrounding tissue is teased away from the nerve to form a path for the placement of the simulator cuff.
6. Nerve stimulator lead cuff is placed around the inclusion branches of XII. The corner of the outer flap of the cuff is held with a right-angled dissector and positioned beneath the nerve. The outer flap is gently positioned past the nerve so the shorter, superior flap of the cuff wraps on to all isolated branches of the nerve. The right-angled dissector is then released, allowing both flaps to completely wrap around nerve XII. Ensure both flaps of the cuff are free from adhesions or other trapped tissue (Fig. 2).
7. Pass the anchor of the stimulator cuff under digastric tendon. Secure the anchor to the anterior belly of the digastric muscle by placing two 3-0 silk sutures on RB-1 needle and positioning the suture into the grooves on the anchor. Place moist gauze into the surgical site and proceed to the next incision.
8. IPG pocket incision is carried through the skin and subcutaneous tissue and superficial to the pectoralis major fascia. Bluntly dissect superficially to the fascia and avoid vessels. The pocket should be approximately 4 cm deep and should be oriented to support arm motions and daily activities. Place moist gauze into the surgical site and proceed to the next incision.
9. Inferolateral chest incision is carried through the skin, subcutaneous tissue, and either through or working between the anterior serratus muscle fibers. Surgeons must avoid the intercostal neurovascular bundle located beneath each rib. A dissector is used to make a small opening through the external intercostal fibers until the internal intercostal fibers are visualized. A narrow malleable retractor is tunneled 6 cm between the internal and external intercostal muscles to accommodate the sensor lead. Surgeons must be cautious to not proceed through the internal intercostal muscle and violate the plural space. The sensor lead is positioned facing the internal intercostal muscle by only grasping the tapered, honeycomb area to prevent damage to the sensor lead. Maintain sensor lead parallel to the ribs. Secure the fixed anchor to the fascia with four 2-0 silk sutures (Fig. 3).
10. Assemble the tunneling device by screwing the collet and sleeve apparatus to the shaft. Prebend the shaft and guide the tunneling device in the subcutaneous plane from the inferolateral chest incision site to the IPG pocket incision site. Stay superficial to the pectoralis major and avoid involvement of breast tissue. Once the tip of the tunneling device has reached the destination incision, attach the opposite end of the sensor lead into the collet of the tunneling device and lock into place by gently sliding the sleeve. Pull the tunneling device from the destination incision site, which results in positioning of the opposite end of the sensor lead at the IPG site. Release the sensor lead from the tunneling device by sliding the sleeve. Secure the movable anchor to the fascia at the interolateral incision site with four 2-0 silk sutures and provide excess sensor lead length between the fixed and movable anchors to accommodate for chest motion (Fig. 4).

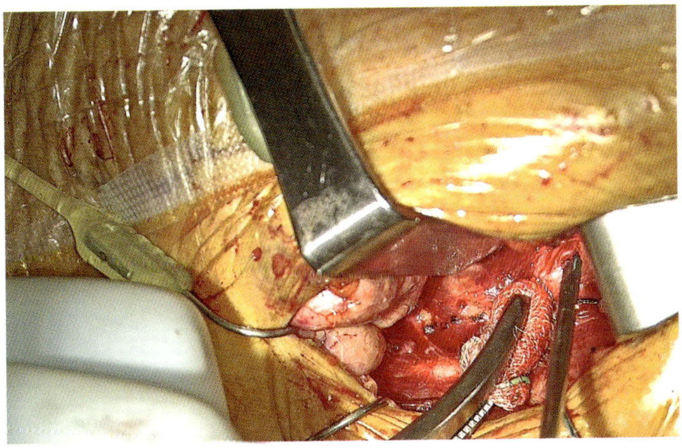

Fig. 1 Nerve test.

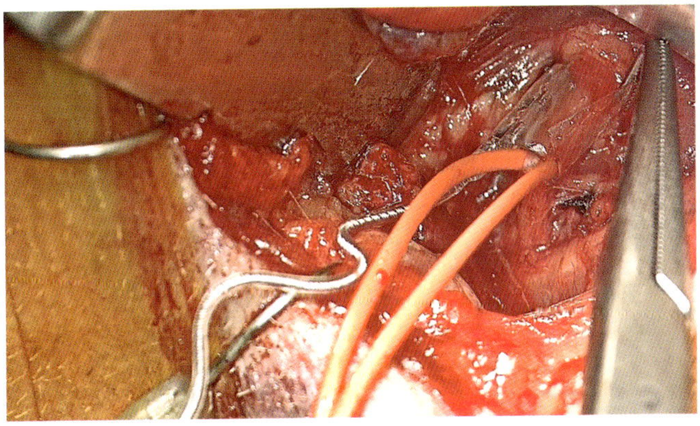

Fig. 2 Stimulation cuff.

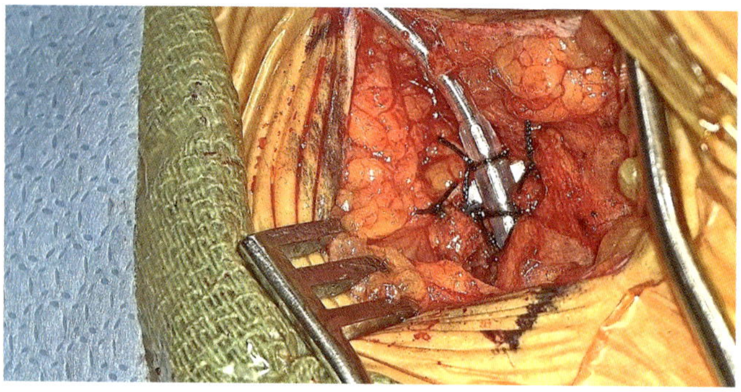

Fig. 3 Chest lead.

11. Prebend the shaft to conform to the neck curvature and pass the tunneling device in the subcutaneous or subplatysmal plane from the neck incision to the IPG incision site. Once the tip of the tunneling device has reached the destination incision, attach the opposite end of the stimulation lead into the collet of the tunneling device and lock into place by gently sliding the sleeve. Pull the tunneling device from the destination incision site, which results in positioning of the opposite end of the stimulation lead at the IPG site. Release the stimulation lead from the tunneling device by sliding the sleeve.
12. Secure the sensor and stimulator leads in the IPG generator by first placing the sensor lead in the inferior port. Insert wrench in the distal screw and fully seat the screw until it protrudes beyond the distal connector block. Perform tug test on the lead to ensure it is secured in the IPG. Next insert wrench in the proximal screw and full seat the strew until it protrudes beyond the distal connector block. Repeat the same steps for the stimulation lead, which is placed in the superior port.
13. Ensure that the engraved side of the IPG is facing outward. Loosely wrap excess lead length around the IPG and insert the IPG with the lead into the tissue pocket. Place two 2-0 silk sutures on SH needle air knots in the pectoralis major fascia at the medial edge of the incision and pass through the same suture hole on the IPG, forming a balance V-shaped sling. This prevents the subcutaneous IPG from wandering and minimizing discomfort.
14. Verify sensing lead function by introducing telemetry head through sterile sleeve and place over the IPG. Assess sensor waveform for up to 30 seconds for clear rise and fall of waveform, denoting respiratory inspiration and expiration phases. Ensure the cuff flaps are encircling entire nerve and visually verify tongue protrusion by running test amplitude 1.0 V down to 0.5 V and below in default configuration. Program therapy off and configure amplitude to 0.0 V.
15. Close all incisions in layers and place pressure dressing material with Telfa and fluffs.

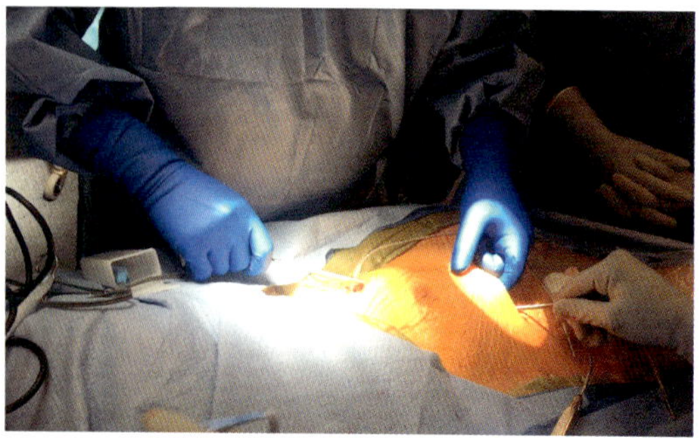

Fig. 4 Tunnel.

Potential complications

USA therapy studies have demonstrated high level of success and low complication rates.[9,16] Overall, a majority of the adverse events were reported soon postoperatively with a high rate of resolution past the first year. The complications can be categorized due to the surgical procedure of implantable device.

Surgical procedure

Adverse events related to the surgical procedure include discomfort at the incision site or away from the incision site, tongue weakness, throat discomfort due to intubation, headaches, hematoma, and mild infection. Most of the adverse events resolve within the first year. The 5-year STAR trial reported 1 patient out of 126 with persistent discomfort at the incision site, with resolution of the other adverse events.[16]

Device related

Adverse events due to the implantable device include discomfort due to electrical stimulation, tongue abrasion, dry mouth, mechanical pain, functionality complaint, and infection. According to the 5-year STAR trial,[16] the most common adverse event was discomfort due to electrical stimulation, which occurred 81 times in the first year. Tongue abrasion was the next most common adverse event that reduced to 2 occurrences at 5 years. Tongue abrasion due to UAS can also be treated by temporarily wearing occlusal mouthguard during sleep. This event diminished to 5 occurrences at 5 years after reprogramming and acclimation. One patient had 2 revision procedures to reposition the neurostimulator and the sensing lead due to discomfort. One patient underwent stimulation lead repositioning due to unfavorable tongue movement and to improve therapy response. Four participants had insulation material failure and underwent replacement of both leads.

Pearls and pitfalls

1. Careful selection of patients for UAS based on the diagnostic, inclusion, and exclusion criteria.
2. Multidisciplinary team consisting of sleep medicine and surgical service needed to optimize patient selection and therapy success.
3. Due to diathermy concerns, use only bipolar cautery and avoid monopolar cautery. Electrical current can damage the UAS device.
4. Use strict sterile techniques and do not use drains to minimize infection risk.
5. If NIM provides unclear signals, then surgeon must rely on other techniques to evaluate the targeted airway.
   a. Direct visualization of the main trunk and course of the hypoglossal nerve.
   b. Direct visualization of the contraction of the HG muscle when stimulating the HG branch from the hypoglossal

nerve. Mixed activation of the HG and GG indicates that the final l-XII
HG branch is in the cuff and must be excluded.

6. Do not place pressure or bend the collet when passing the leads because this may lead to breakage of the collet.

Immediate postoperative care

1. Obtain postoperative radiograph to document implant placement and rule-out pneumothorax (anterior-posterior for all 3 implant sites and lateral for stimulator lead, which includes chin-to-cervical vertebrae)
2. Plan for same-day discharge or overnight observation per surgeon discretion.
3. Place arm in sling on the same side as IPG pocket to restrict range of motion of arm and shoulder for days 1 to 2.
4. Normal diet and light activities after day 1.

Rehabilitation and recovery

1. One week post–implant placement:
   a. Surgical evaluation and suture removal. Pain and swelling should begin to resolve 7 days to 10 days postoperatively.
   b. Resume activities of daily living.
   c. Avoid strenuous activities that require arm/shoulder motion and no shoulder abduction greater than 90°.
2. One month post–implant placement:
   a. Resume vigorous activities with appropriate protections for IPG and leads.
   b. Activate device and teach patient how to use remote and device at home. Patient uses therapy at home for a few months for acclimation and up-titration of simulation level as tolerated.
3. Two to 3 months post implant placement:
   a. Optimize nerve stimulator settings during PSG with presence of sleep medicine and Inspire Medical Systems technicians.
4. Every 5 months to 12 months post–implant placement:
   a. Routine checks of simulator and surgical sites.

Clinical results in the literature

Neuromuscular stimulation of the hypoglossal nerve and genioglossus muscle is an effective physiologic treatment of the upper airway. The UAS devices have evolved over the years to provide a more precise target of the inclusion branches of the hypoglossal nerve to treat the retroglossal and retropalatal areas of the airway. Inspire Medical Systems has obtained Food and Drug Administration approval for a UAS device. The 5-year results from the STAR trial in 2018 have shown significant improvements in PSG measures, where the median AHI has decreased from 29.3 to 6.2, and quality-of-life outcomes, where the FOSQ scores increased from 14.6 to 18.7, ESS scores decreased from 11 to 6, and no or soft snoring scores increased from 17% to 90%.[16] The STAR trial has also established precision surgical care in using DISE to exclude nonresponders and in utilization of NIM monitoring to identify hypoglossal nerve branches of tongue protrusive muscles. Multiple studies have shown consistent AHI reduction and UAS therapy adherence.[18–20]

A model-based projection based on the STAR trial demonstrated the long-term health outcomes and incremental cost-effectiveness of UAS compared with no treatment. UAS substantially reduced clinical events, such as 10-year reductions in cardiovascular events by 25% to 37%, and reduced motor vehicle collisions projected over a patient's lifetime and resulted in gain in total quality-adjusted life expectancy of 1.7 years.[21] Untreated obstructive sleep apnea (OSA) syndrome can lead to increased cardiovascular disease, stroke, metabolic disease, excessive daytime sleepiness, workplace errors, traffic accidents and death, which are associated with significant economic burden.[22] Although UAS is less cost effective than PAP therapy in treating OSA, patients who remain untreated after PAP therapy trial would lead to a significant economic burden on society. As a result, the short-term costs associated with UAS should be accepted, with the potential significant long-term savings with reduction in comorbidities, traffic accidents, and loss of workdays.

A study out of Cleveland Clinic showed that although both traditional surgery and UAS are effective treatments for patients with moderate to severe OSA with CPAP intolerance, UAS is curative in normalizing the AHI to less than 5 in a majority of patients.[23] For patients who underwent UAS, mean AHI decreased significantly from 38.9 ± 12.5 to 4.5 ± 4.8, and all patients achieved an AHI less than 20 postimplant, with 65% (13/20) with an AHI less than or equal to 5. For patients who underwent traditional airway surgery, mean AHI decreased from 40.3 ± 12.4 to 28.8 ± 25.4. Additional studies are needed that compare the effectiveness of various sleep surgical procedures with the UAS.

Patients with multilevel obstruction may be treated with traditional Stanford protocol phase 1 consisting of nasal, palatal, and tongue base surgery; MMA, or UAS. DISE is a critical diagnostic tool in aiding surgeons in selection of the appropriate surgical intervention as the primary treatment.[24] Each of these surgical techniques also may serve as and adjunctive therapy to further treat residual or relapse OSA. DISE evaluation of patients who have recently undergone MMA and of patients presenting with long-term OSA relapse has shown minimal velum and lateral pharyngeal wall collapse.[25] As a result, based on the current inclusion criteria for UAS, it is highly likely that patients previously successfully treated with MMA who later present with relapse would be good candidates for hypoglossal stimulation.[26]

Summary

Patients with OSA who are intolerant to PAP therapy can be treated effectively with UAS. DISE is an essential evaluation step to exclude patients with retropalatal concentric collapse. Preparation of CN XII and determination of functional breakpoint to exclude the lateral XII branches and include the medial XII branches is critical to optimize surgical success. Studies have shown up to 5-year follow-up with hypoglossal nerve stimulation providing improvements in outcome measures, such as quality of life, ESS, snoring, and PSG values.

References

1. Dempsey JA, Veasey SC, Morgan BJ, et al. Pathophysiology of sleep apnea. Physiol Rev 2010;90(1):47–112.
2. Young T, Finn L, Peppard PE, et al. Sleep disordered breathing and mortality: eighteen-year follow-up of the Wisconsin sleep cohort. Sleep 2008;31(8):1071–8.

3. Wolk R, Somers VK. Sleep and the metabolic syndrome. Exp Physiol 2007;92(1):67–78.
4. Einhorn D, Stewart DA, Erman MK, et al. Prevalence of sleep apnea in a population of adults with type 2 diabetes mellitus. Endocr Pract 2007;13(4):355–62.
5. Caples SM, Rowley JA, Prinsell JR, et al. Surgical modifications of the upper airway for obstructive sleep apnea in adults: a systematic review and meta-analysis. Sleep 2010;33(10): 1396–407.
6. Holty JE, Guilleminault C. Maxillomandibular advancement for the treatment of obstructive sleep apnea: a systematic review and meta-analysis. Sleep Med Rev 2010;14(5):287–97.
7. Friedman M, Jacobowitz O, Hwang MS, et al. Targeted hypoglossal nerve stimulation for the treatment of obstructive sleep apnea: six-month results. Laryngoscope 2016;126(11):2618–23.
8. Mwenge GB, Rombaux P, Lengele B, et al. Hypoglossal nerve stimulation for obstructive sleep apnea. Prog Neurol Surg 2015;29: 94–105.
9. Van de Heyning PH, Badr MS, Baskin JZ, et al. Implanted upper airway stimulation device for obstructive sleep apnea. Laryngoscope 2012;122(7):1626–33.
10. Schwartz AR, Bennett ML, Smith PL, et al. Therapeutic electrical stimulation of the hypoglossal nerve in obstructive sleep apnea. Arch Otolaryngol Head Neck Surg 2001;127(10):1216–23.
11. Goding GS, Tesfayesus W, Kezirian EJ. Hypoglossal nerve stimulation and airway changes under fluoroscopy. Otolaryngol Head Neck Surg 2012;146(6):1017–22.
12. Safiruddin F, Vanderveken OM, de Vries N, et al. Effect of upper-airway stimulation for obstructive sleep apnoea on airway dimensions. Eur Respir J 2015;45(1):129–38.
13. Vanderveken OM, Maurer JT, Hohenhorst W, et al. Evaluation of drug-induced sleep endoscopy as a patient selection tool for implanted upper airway stimulation for obstructive sleep apnea. J Clin Sleep Med 2013;9(5):433–8.
14. Kezirian EJ, Hohenhorst W, de Vries N. Drug-induced sleep endoscopy: the VOTE classification. Eur Arch Otorhinolaryngol 2011;268(8):1233–6.
15. Strohl KP, Baskin J, Lance C, et al. Origins of and implementation concepts for upper airway stimulation therapy for obstructive sleep apnea. Respir Investig 2016;54(4):241–9.
16. Woodson BT, Strohl KP, Soose RJ, et al. Upper airway stimulation for obstructive sleep apnea: 5-year outcomes. Otolaryngol Head Neck Surg 2018;159(1):194–202.
17. Yegїn Y, Çelik M, Kaya KH, et al. Comparison of drug-induced sleep endoscopy and Müller's maneuver in diagnosing obstructive sleep apnea using the VOTE classification system. Braz J Otorhinolaryngol 2017;83(4):445–50.
18. Huntley C, Kaffenberger T, Doghramji K, et al. Upper airway stimulation for treatment of obstructive sleep apnea: an evaluation and comparison of outcomes at two academic centers. J Clin Sleep Med 2017;13(9):1075–9.
19. Hofauer B, Steffen A, Knopf A, et al. Patient experience with upper airway stimulation in the treatment of obstructive sleep apnea. Sleep Breath 2018 [Epub ahead of print].
20. Boon M, Huntley C, Steffen A, et al. Upper airway stimulation for obstructive sleep apnea: results from the ADHERE registry. Otolaryngol Head Neck Surg 2018;159(2):379–85.
21. Pietzsch JB, Liu S, Garner AM, et al. Long-term cost-effectiveness of upper airway stimulation for the treatment of obstructive sleep apnea: a model-based projection based on the STAR trial. Sleep 2015;38(5):735–44.
22. Knauert M, Naik S, Gillespie MB, et al. Clinical consequences and economic costs of untreated obstructive sleep apnea syndrome. World J Otorhinolaryngol Head Neck Surg 2015;1(1):17–27.
23. Shah J, Russell JO, Waters T, et al. Uvulopalatopharyngoplasty vs CN XII stimulation for treatment of obstructive sleep apnea: a single institution experience. Am J Otolaryngol 2018;39(3): 266–70.
24. Huntley C, Chou D, Doghramji K, et al. Preoperative drug induced sleep endoscopy improves the surgical approach to treatment of obstructive sleep apnea. Ann Otol Rhinol Laryngol 2017;126(6): 478–82.
25. Liu SY, Huon LK, Iwasaki T, et al. Efficacy of maxillomandibular advancement examined with drug-induced sleep endoscopy and computational fluid dynamics airflow modeling. Otolaryngol Head Neck Surg 2016;154(1):189–95.
26. Liu SY, Riley RW. Continuing the original Stanford sleep surgery protocol from upper airway reconstruction to upper airway stimulation: our first successful case. J Oral Maxillofac Surg 2017;75(7): 1514–8.

Transoral Robotic Surgery for the Tongue Base

Ghali E. Ghali, DDS, MD, FACS, FRCS(Ed) , Andrew T. Meram, DDS, MD*

KEYWORDS

• Transoral • Robotic • Base of tongue • Sleep apnea

KEY POINTS

- Obstructive sleep apnea-hypopnea syndrome (OSAHS) is a common disorder that affects 2% to 4% of men and 1% to 2% of women between the ages of 30 and 69 years, and is increasingly becoming recognized as a major health problem.
- Surgery with transoral robotic surgery (TORS) offers significant advantages compared with traditional open surgical approaches to the pharynx.
- TORS allows for high-quality endoscopic optics for improved visualization with three-dimensional depth perception and robotic instrumentation.
- The chief indications include a failed trial of continuous positive airway pressure, with polysomnographic evidence of moderate to severe OSAHS, in addition to daytime somnolence as documented through the Epworth Sleepiness Scale, with evidence of retrolingual collapse from a prominent base of tongue and/or prominent lingual tonsillar tissue.
- The rate of success, defined as 50% reduction of preoperative apnea-hypopnea index (AHI) and an AHI less than 20, is achieved in up to 76.6% of patients.

Introduction

Several surgical procedures have been developed to address tongue base obstruction, including tissue debulking procedures (midline glossectomy, radiofrequency ablation) and tissue repositioning (tongue suspension, genioglossal advancement, maxillomandibular advancement), each with varying results.[1,2] The traditional external tongue base approach provides excellent exposure, although the potential for morbidity is significant. Minimally invasive transoral techniques include radiofrequency ablation, laser-assisted oropharyngeal surgery, submucosal minimally invasive lingual excision, and coblation endoscopic lingual lightening.[3] There is limited evidence of their long-term efficacy, and suboptimal transoral access remains an issue. Base of tongue collapse is, therefore, challenging to address secondary to difficult surgical access and visualization along with uncertainty with regard to the volume of tissue that can be safely excised.[1] Thus, there existed a critical need to improve surgical treatment of patients with obstructive sleep apnea-hypopnea syndrome (OSAHS) through either a shift in treatment paradigm or technological advances.

Robot-assisted technology was investigated as a means to overcome the surgical limitation associated with current technologies. Transoral robotic surgery (TORS) for resection of oropharyngeal and supraglottic neoplasms using the da Vinci Surgical System (Intuitive Surgical, Sunnyvale, CA) was pioneered by Weinstein and O'Malley in 2006.[4,5] In 2009, the US Food and Drug Administration (FDA) approved TORS for benign and malignant lesions of the tongue base.[1,6] This technique was extended to transoral resection of the base of tongue and supraglottoplasty in patients with OSAHS by Vicini and colleagues[7] in 2009, and in 2014 the FDA approved TORS procedures for benign base-of-tongue resection procedures after its safety and feasibility in patients with OSAHS were shown.[1,6,8] Since then, it has been shown to be an effective treatment option for both solely base-of-tongue procedures and when combined with multilevel surgery. TORS has the ability to overcome the issues with surgical access that had previously hampered surgical treatment options. The robot system allows for high-quality endoscopic optics for improved visualization with three-dimensional (3D) depth perception and robotic instrumentation.[5,8,9] The instruments have 6 degrees of freedom and 90° of articulation, which provides superior dexterity and precision. At this time, it is estimated that more than 450 TORS procedures for OSAHS have been performed throughout the world.[10]

Indications

The chief indication for surgery in OSAHS is that the patient has failed a trial of continuous positive airway pressure (CPAP) either because of noncompliance or inability to tolerate the device. Typically, the patient should have polysomnographic evidence of moderate to severe OSAHS in addition to daytime somnolence as documented through the Epworth Sleepiness Scale. For TORS-specific surgery, patients should have evidence of retrolingual collapse from a prominent base of tongue and/or prominent lingual tonsillar tissue,[6,8] which is determined

Disclosure Statement: The authors have nothing to disclose.
Department of Oral & Maxillofacial Surgery/Head & Neck Surgery, Louisiana State University Health Sciences Center – Shreveport, 1501 Kings Highway, Shreveport, LA 71103, USA
* Corresponding author.
E-mail address: ameram@lsuhsc.edu

Atlas Oral Maxillofacial Surg Clin N Am 27 (2019) 59–66
1061-3315/19/
https://doi.org/10.1016/j.cxom.2018.11.002

either by awake nasopharyngoscopy or drug-induced sleep endoscopy.[8] Most patients are overweight men, but patients with a preoperative body mass index (BMI) less than 30 kg/m^2 are preferred. Mouth opening measured as interincisive distance of 25 mm or more is a prerequisite for sufficient exposure.[7] The aim of these surgical procedures is to enlarge the airway space and/or increase the muscular tension around the retroglossal region by reducing soft tissue volume or by altering the facial skeleton framework.[11]

Contraindications

Contraindications for TORS are classified as patient compliance, patient anatomy, and medical comorbidities. If the patient is compliant with CPAP, or in those who have not yet tried CPAP, surgical intervention is discouraged. A degree of trismus or limited mobility of the neck may make the base of tongue inaccessible. Significant micrognathia and macroglossia may also limit the exposure for TORS procedures.[8] Dynamic compression of the lateral airway from soft tissue is a relative contraindication because TORS essentially addresses only anterior-posterior collapse of the airway.[8] An American Society of Anesthesiologists (ASA) score greater than 2 with particular reference to significant or unstable cardiovascular disease or the need for anticoagulation must be treated with caution. Patients with any degree of dysphagia (unless secondary to lingual tonsillar hypertrophy), swallowing complaints, or psychiatric illnesses should also not be considered for TORS.[6]

Relevant anatomy

The base of the tongue has a rich vascular supply from the lingual artery. Significant vessels are located laterally and inferiorly. The average length of the lingual artery as visualized by computed tomography angiography is 101.24 $\pm$ 16.99 mm.[12] The dorsal lingual artery is the major branch that arises from the lingual artery, usually below the hyoglossus muscle. At the level of the hyoid bone, it is located above it and medial to the hypoglossal nerve. Inferiorly located, with regard to the artery, lies the lingual vein, which, in turn, accompanies the hypoglossal nerve, which is invisible preoperatively and intraoperatively.[8,12] The medial region of the tongue base is without major vessels. There are numerous small branches from the lingual artery approaching the midline. These branches can be used as a safe plane to remind the surgeon to be extremely careful when dissecting deeper.[13]

The foramen caecum linguae is an important anatomic landmark for midline partial glossectomy surgery. Anatomically, the foramen caecum linguae is located at the one-third middle and posterior junction.[12] The average distance from the foramen caecum to the hypoglossal/lingual artery neurovascular bundle was 1.66 cm in a cadaver study, and 1.68 cm in a study using computed tomography angiography.[4] The average distance between 2 lingual arteries at the foramen caecum of the tongue was 27.78 $\pm$ 6.57 mm, and the distance to the surface of the tongue was 29.27 $\pm$ 5.39 mm.[4,12] Therefore, 15 mm and 20 mm are used as the surgical functional zone based on the average distance and 95% confidence interval for the distance between bilateral lingual arteries and arteries to the tongue surface, respectively.[12]

Lingual tonsils are parts of the Waldeyer ring along with the palatine tonsils, adenoids, tubal tonsils, and lateral pharyngeal bands. Lingual tonsils are situated at the base of tongue and bounded by the epiglottis posteriorly, circumvallate papillae anteriorly, and tonsillar pillars bilaterally.[14]

Surgical technique

Patient preparation and positioning

An appropriate mouth gag is chosen to provide adequate exposure to the anatomic structures without compromising the workspace necessary for the robotic arms and instruments. The authors use the Davis Meyer (Karl Storz, El Segundo, CA) retractor, which includes multiple tongue blades of different lengths. The surgery is performed with the da Vinci Surgical System (Intuitive Surgical, Sunnyvale, CA). The required robotic instrumentation includes the high-definition camera and the EndoWrist instruments (Intuitive Surgical, Sunnyvale, CA). The binocular camera provides magnification of up to 10 times, which results in a 3D high-definition image that allows easy identification of vessels and nerves. It is available in 12-mm and 8-mm diameter scopes, both of which provide excellent optics while providing adequate working space in the mouth. Two 5-mm articulated EndoWrist instrument arms are typically used. These instrument arms provide 180° of articulation and 540° of rotation, tremor filtration, and amplitude scaling, and allow bimanual tissue manipulation in multiple planes. Typically, a 5-mm Maryland forceps is placed in one arm and the spatula-tip monopolar cautery in the other for dissection and coagulation (Fig. 1).

It is imperative to have ready sufficient overhead lighting, a Yankauer suction, an additional cautery device, appropriate-length forceps, hemostats, Metzenbaum scissors, and other basic soft tissue instruments (Fig. 2). The patient gurney should

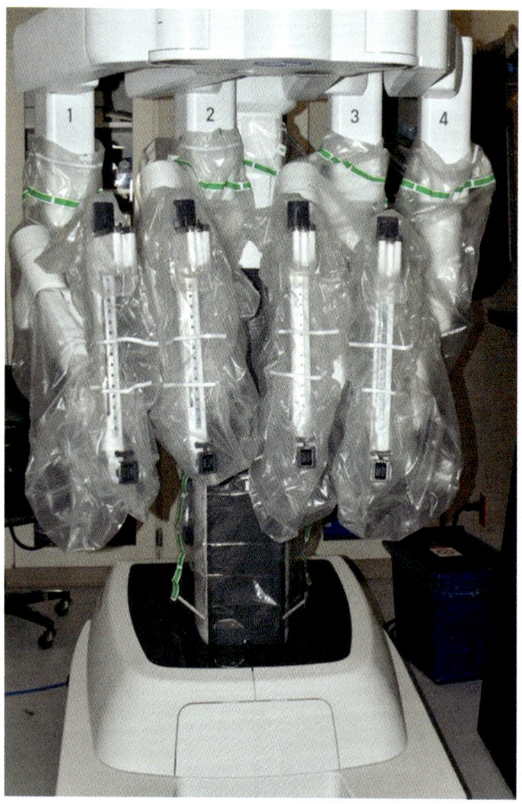

Fig. 1 Standard drape for Da Vinci Robotic surgery.

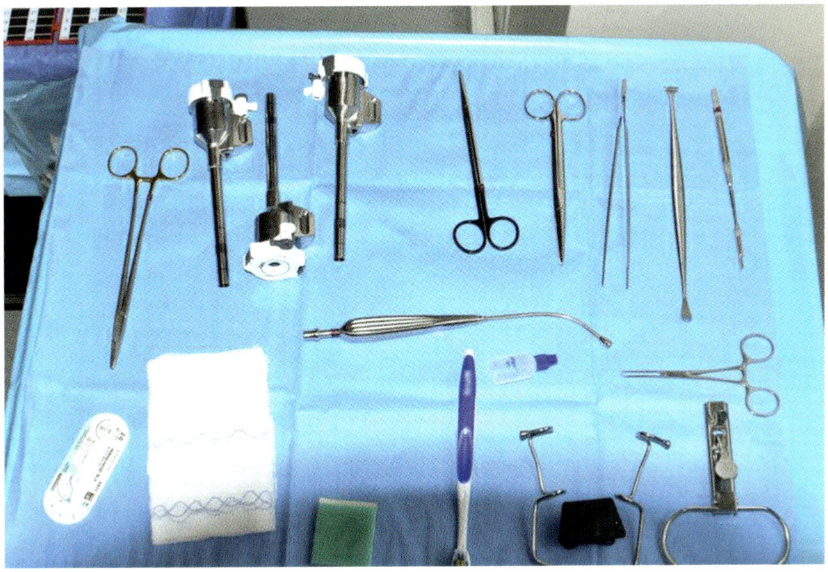

Fig. 2 Operative tray instrument set-up

be centered with the surgeon console approximately 1.8 to 2.1 m (6 to 7 feet) away. The surgeon console should be situated on the same side of the operating table as the assisting surgeon to allows for easier communication between the assistant and the console surgeon. The anesthesia cart is placed at the foot of the bed (patient's head is turned 180° from anesthesia) and the assistant is seated at the head of the patient to provide suctioning and assistance with cauterization. The scrub nurse stands alongside the patient cart opposite the robotic console. Difficult-airway equipment, including a fiberoptic endoscope or GlideScope (Verathon Medical, Bothell, WA), must be readily available.

The primary surgeon is seated at the robotic console, which is typically in close proximity to the operating room table. The console affords a 3D view of the surgical field and allows manipulation of the 2 robotic arms and the camera https://www.intuitive.com/en/products-and-services/da-vinci. The surgical assistant supports the primary surgeon by retracting tissues, creating a smoke-free environment, and suctioning blood to aid visualization. As needed, the assistant helps with adjusting the robotic arms and camera to prevent collisions, as well as facilitate hemostasis. There is an integrated microphone-loudspeaker system inbuilt in the robotic system that aids communication between the primary and assistant surgeon. The surgical scrub aids in passing instruments and providing equipment as needed but may also provide assistance with suctioning. It is imperative that the surgical scrub is familiar with the TORS setup to aid in decreasing both setup and operative time. The assistant surgeon and the surgical scrub can see a two-dimensional representation of the surgeon's view on the slave monitor, which is attached to the robot in the da Vinci S HD model and to the control tower–vision cart in the Si model.

The patient is positioned supine and the upper airway is anesthetized with topical lidocaine. The patient is then intubated with a nasotracheal tube and the operating table is turned 180° from the anesthesia cart (Fig. 3). A 2-0 silk stitch is placed in the anterior portion of the tongue to assist in retraction and positioning of the tongue. The mouth gag is placed to provide adequate exposure of the base of the tongue. At this point, the surgical bed is lowered to the lowest position possible. A Mayo stand without the accompanying tray should be placed over the patient's head so that the curved end of the retractor blade can be connected to the Mayo stand, and the stand elevated to help hyperextend the neck (Figs. 4 and 5). The robotic patient side cart is wheeled to the patient's head so that the base of the cart is approximately on a 30° angle with the base of the surgical bed. The robotic base may come from either the left or right side depending on the room setup.

The 3 robotic arms are positioned in a triangular format. The camera is placed in the center arm and the grasping instrument and cutting instrument are placed on the side arms depending on which side of the base of the tongue is addressed first (Fig. 6). The instruments are inserted into the patient's mouth so that the apices of the instruments meet in the operative area. The base of the tongue is viewed using the 30° 12-mm camera, facing up. The Maryland 5-mm forceps is placed in the left arm and the spatula-tip cautery in the right arm.

Surgical procedure

Standard fire precautions are taken, the Fio_2(fraction of inspired oxygen) should be kept less than 30%, and suction Bovie and Hemoclips are available on the back table should they be necessary. The surgeon is seated at the console. Landmarks should be identified: the circumvallate papillae, foramen caecum, vallecula, and epiglottis. The borders of the right lingual tonsil are identified and marked with cautery to outline the resection margins. The margins extend superiorly from the sulcus terminalis, laterally from the glossopharyngeal sulcus, and inferiorly to the glossoepiglottic sulcus (Fig. 7). In some patients, it is difficult to visualize the epiglottis at the start of the procedure, but it should be seen as the dissection progresses. The procedure is begun by removing the lymphatic tissue from the base of the tongue first on the right side and then on the left. Dissection is performed just posterior from the circumvallate papillae, down into the vallecula, and across to the base of the epiglottis, dissecting the lymphatic tissue off of the underlying musculature. The inferior limit of the surgical

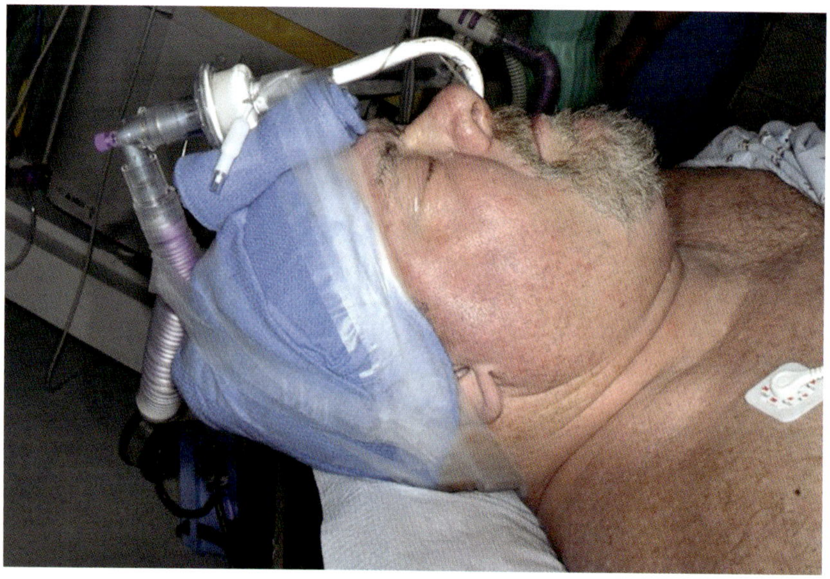

Fig. 3 Standard head-wrap with nasal RAE secured to head-wrap.

bed is recognized by a bluish color of the vallecular mucosa. It is often easier to perform a midline split of the lymphatic tissue from the foramen caecum down to the base of the epiglottis, and remove the right and left sides separately. The procedure is then repeated on the left side. Hemostasis is obtained during the dissection and great care is taken laterally to avoid the lingual artery and its branches. Once the lymphatic tissue has been removed, the procedure is repeated, removing a layer of muscle across the tongue base (up to 10 mm), right and then left side, and if necessary an additional strip of muscle (up to 5 mm) may be removed in the midline only, to avoid injury to the lingual nerve (Fig. 8). The final amount of tissue resected is measured right after the resection by immersing the tissue in saline and measuring the amount of saline displaced inside a 120-mL sterile specimen cup. The average amount of tissue removed is approximately 10 mL, depending on the individual, and studies have shown a trend toward the amount of tissue removed and success. Removal of less than 7 mL of tissue is likely insufficient for success, and greater than 20 mL of tissue removal is often not needed.[4,6,10] Hemostatic agents are usually not necessary. It is of paramount importance to use the midline of the tongue base as the point of reference to minimize the risk to the hypoglossal nerve, lingual artery, and lingual neural branches. Patients are usually extubated in the operating room and observed overnight in a monitored bed. If the airway is deemed to be too tenuous, the surgeon may prefer to leave the patient intubated or perform a tracheostomy.

Potential complications

The overall frequency of early postoperative major medical complications after surgery for the management of OSAHS is

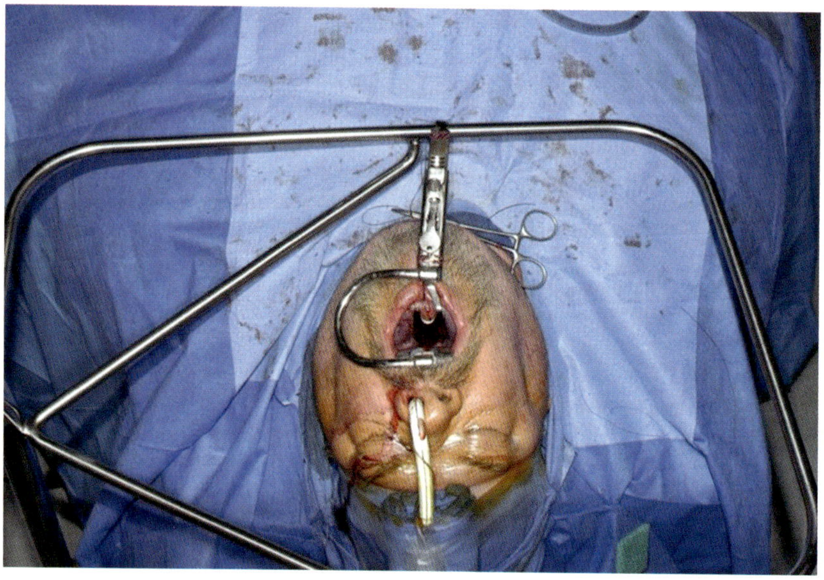

Fig. 4 Overhead view of Crow-Davis retractor attached to Mayo stand.

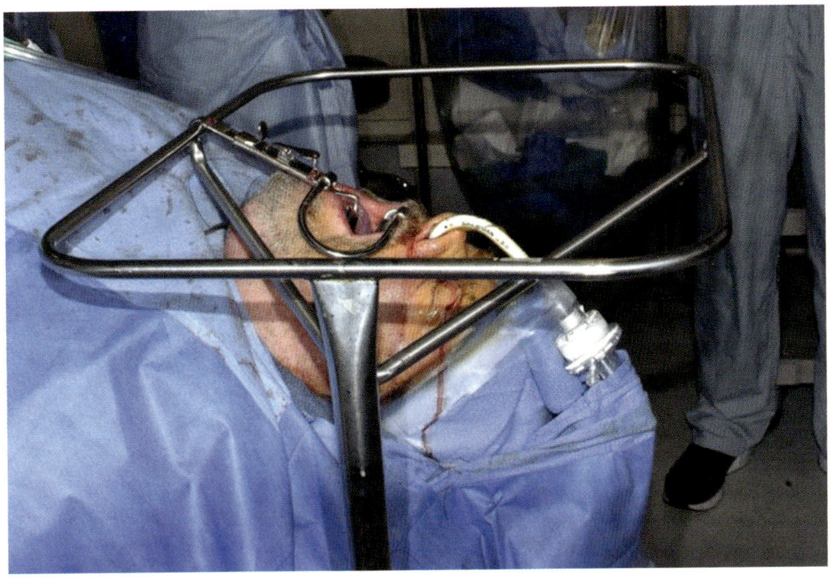

Fig. 5 Lateral view of Crow-Davis retractor attached to Mayo stand.

low (2.2%).[15] With respect to TORS specifically, the most common complications include temporary dysphagia (5.1%), dehydration (4.8%), hypogeusia, and limited late bleeding (4.1%).[6,7] Patients often complain of difficulty swallowing and taste disturbance, both of which usually resolve by 2 to 3 weeks but can last longer or (rarely) be permanent. Late bleeding is seen in 3% to 4% of cases (similar to tonsillectomy postoperative bleeding) and usually occurs 2 to 3 weeks postoperatively.[2,8] This bleeding is often self-limited, but requires intervention in some cases. Occasionally patients complain of temporary tongue numbness from paresis of the lingual nerve caused by pressure on the tongue from the mouth gag. This numbness usually resolves in 2 to 4 weeks. Limiting the amount of time the mouth gag is in place and opened helps to avoid this problem, because patients in suspension for less than 45 minutes are less likely to develop these complications.[7,8] Other potential complications include tooth or lip injury, transient pharyngeal or supraglottic edema, and pharyngeal scarring. More severe complications include intraoperative bleeding from injury to the lingual artery or one of its branches, which may require opening the neck to gain control; loss of the airway; death; and paralysis of the hypoglossal nerve, which has not been reported. In a study by Glazer and colleagues[16] involving 293 TORS procedures for OSAHS, the complication rate was 20.7%. In a series of 243 TORS procedures for OSAHS, Vicini and colleagues[13] reported transient and mild hypogeusia as the most common complication (14.2%) and a 5.0% bleed rate (2.9% late bleeding and self-limited, 1.7% requiring surgical intervention, and a 0.4% rate of significant intraoperative hemorrhage).

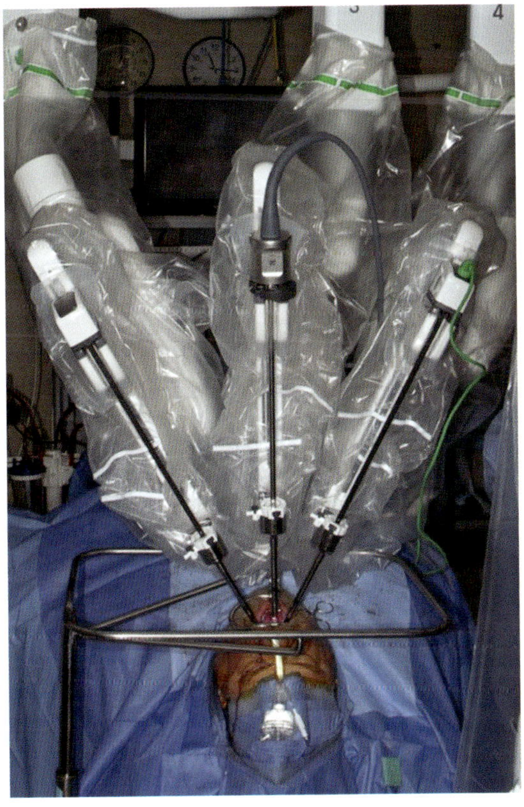

Fig. 6 Triangulation of da Vinci arms for surgery.

The risk of postoperative bleeding has a bimodal distribution, with one peak within hours of surgery and the second within 7 to 10 days of surgery.[8,16] Patients must be advised of this risk and told to present to an emergency department immediately should any bleeding occur. This bleeding, as with routine posttonsillectomy hemorrhage, is treated conservatively or operatively, depending on severity.

Glazer and colleagues[16] studied the factors that correlated with complications. They found that ASA score ($P = .003$) and number of adjunct procedures ($P = .004$) correlated with postoperative complications, whereas age, BMI, apnea-hypopnea index (AHI), lowest oxygen saturation (LSAT), number of comorbidities, and anticoagulation therapy were dissociated.[17] It is our impression that most patients experience mild prolonged dysphagia and globus sensation. A 7-kg (15-pound) weight loss can be expected in the first 2 to 3 weeks postoperatively; however, at 3 months postoperatively, the BMI is likely to have returned to preoperative levels. The most troublesome complaint for patients is the persistent foreign-body sensation that can accompany routine

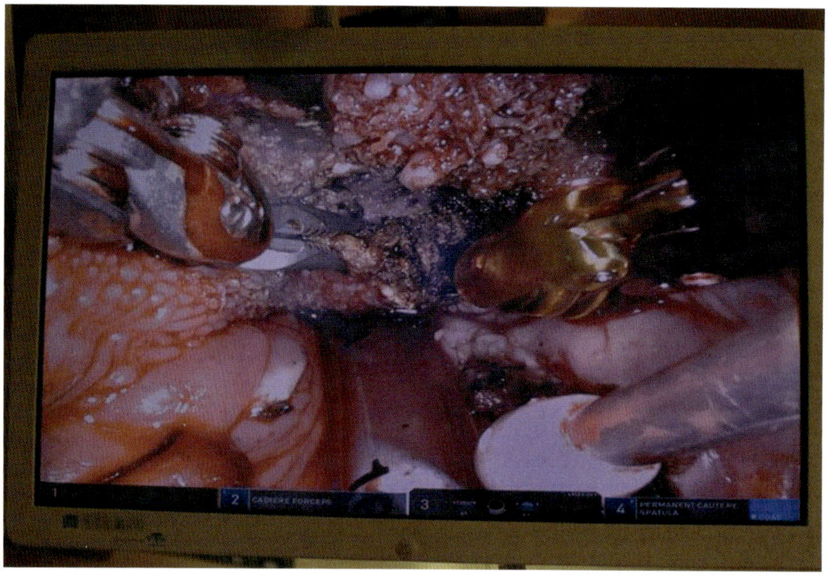

Fig. 7 View of electrocautery instrument removing base of tongue tissue.

swallowing, of which there does not seem to be any correlation with the extent of lingual tonsillectomy or base-of-tongue resection.

Pearls and pitfalls

Surgical treatment of obstruction at the level of the base of tongue has traditionally been challenging because of difficulty in accessing this region. TORS may overcome this limitation by offering improved visualization and surgical access to the base-of-tongue region.[18]

Surgery with TORS offers significant advantages compared with traditional open surgical approaches to the pharynx. A transoral, minimally invasive approach avoids large incisions in the neck, mandibulotomies, pharyngotomies, and the resultant morbidity of the open approaches. Tracheotomy and gastrostomy tube placement is infrequent. TORS provides surgeons with a 3D, high-definition view of the operative field from the perspective of being inside the mouth of the patient. The maneuverable, angled endoscope affords a wide field of vision including around the tongue base. The wristed instruments provide precise bimanual tissue manipulation allowing en bloc excision of oropharyngeal tumors.[19]

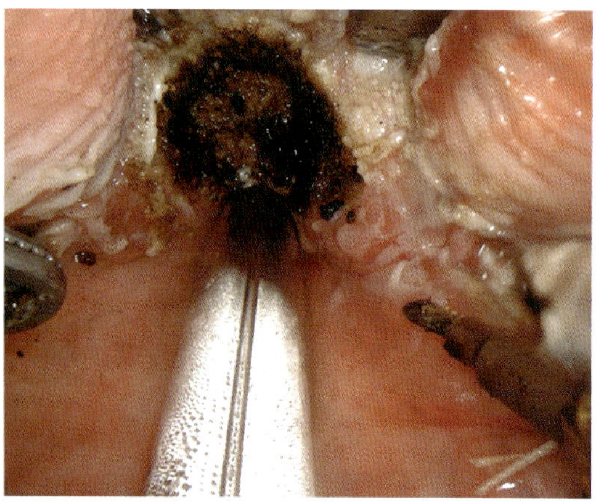

Fig. 8 Resected base of tongue operative site.

Upper airway surgery success is defined as a postoperative AHI of less than 10 events per hour along with at least 50% decrease from the baseline AHI (responders); treatment failure is defined as a postoperative AHI of greater than 10 events per hour and/or a decrease of AHI from baseline less than 50% (nonresponders). The postoperative difference of AHI is defined as the postoperative AHI minus the baseline AHI.[20]

When operating beyond the 1.5-cm boundary from the midline, it is extremely important to increase the magnification to allow the clear visualization of the layer-by-layer cutting of the muscle fibers. Slow and careful dissection should be performed over the lateral base of tongue to identify the dorsal branch of the lingual artery, which needs to be carefully ligated multiple times with clips before dividing.[4]

Immediate postoperative care

Those patients thought to be at significant risk of airway edema based on unfavorable anatomy and extent of tissue resection are left intubated. Otherwise, extubation occurs in the operating room at the end of the procedure. Patients are admitted overnight in an intensive care unit given the potential for bleeding and/or airway edema after TORS tongue-base surgery. Continuous pulse oximetry is recommended. Postoperative intravenous steroids may help with nausea, airway edema, and pain from the inflammatory response. Patients are started on a clear liquid diet that is advanced as tolerated. A feeding tube is optional. A patient-controlled analgesic pump has proved to be useful. The average hospital stay is 2 days. Patients are discharged home when they are tolerating an oral diet with adequate pain control. For most patients this is postoperative day 2. They are sent home with oral antibiotics and a short steroid taper in addition to liquid analgesics.

Rehabilitation and recovery

Patients are followed closely after discharge. Diet is normalized as healing progresses and formal therapist-directed swallowing therapy is used as required. Postoperative polysomnography is performed once healing is complete, usually at least 3 to 6 months following surgery.

Clinical results in the literature

Vicini and colleagues[10] showed that most patients tend to be male (81%), with an average age of 50 ± 12 years. The average BMI was 28.53 ± 3.87, with a range from 20.5 to 40.8. The preoperative AHI was recorded by polysomnography in all patients as well as LSAT. AHI ranged from 5.8 to 112 (average, 43.21 ± 22.60). Average LSAT was 79.20% ± 9.09% (range, 48%–95%). An additional primary parameter was excessive daytime sleepiness as measured by the Epworth Sleepiness Scale score, ranging from 0 to 24 (average, 12.15 ± 5.04). An important preoperative biometric was interincisive distance, with an average value of 4.12 ± 0.64 mm (range, 2.7–5.3 mm).

In terms of length of surgery, the average setup and exposure times were 19.5 ± 10.5 minutes, with a wide range between 10 and 70 minutes. The same large variability was observed (7–60 minutes) in the console time for tongue-base reduction, averaging 26.5 ± 9.2 minutes. When considered as 1 component of a multisite surgery, TORS accounted for an operative time of 55.7 ± 17.1 minutes with an overall operative time of 98.2 ± 49.9 minutes; nonrobotic portions of the procedure nearly double the overall operative time.[10]

TORS allowed a significant volume of safe debulking in the tongue base through the removal of a mixed amount of lymphoid tissue and muscle. The average volume removal (10.29 mL) was lower than the removed tissue in an open approach (25 mL), but higher than in the TORS approach described by Friedman and colleagues[9] (about 3 mL). The open approach is more effective at tissue removal and AHI reduction but has not been widely adopted because of pain, length of hospitalization, dysphagia, and cosmetic sequelae.[10]

Friedman and colleagues[8] reported on 27 patients whose mean AHI dropped from 54.6 ± 21.8 to 18.6 ± 9.1 ($P<.001$) following robotic-assisted midline glossectomy. Vicini and colleagues[13] found that a comparison among preoperative and postoperative parameters showed a significant decrease in postoperative AHI and Epworth Sleepiness Scale, and an increase of the lowest oxygen saturation value. The success rates were defined as 50% reduction of preoperative AHI and an AHI less than 20. The mean rate of failure was 34.4% (29.5%–46.2%). In their meta-analysis, taking into consideration articles about TORS as a part of a multilevel setting, the following can be highlighted: preoperative and postoperative AHI means were, respectively, 46.88 and 20.24, with a mean rate of failure of 36.1% (n = 365). Complications occurred in 21.3% of the patients included in the analysis (n = 820). Transient dysphagia represented the most common complication (7.2%) followed by bleeding (4.2%). Minor complications, such as postoperative pharyngeal edema, were registered in 1% of cases. The complication rate in patients treated with TORS as part of a multilevel intervention was 17.75% (n = 365).[21]

Compelling outcomes in reducing the AHI and daytime sleepiness have been shown in the current body of published studies. The rate of success, defined as 50% reduction of preoperative AHI and an AHI less than 20, is achieved in up to 76.6% of patients, with a range between 53.8% and 83.3%. However, reliable predictors of surgical response remain an area of active research. Lin and colleagues[4] showed that AHI less than 60, BMI less than 30, and no lateral velopharyngeal collapse are independent predictive factors of surgical success. Patients with these characteristics had a success rate of 86.7% after TORS base-of-tongue reduction compared with a 53.8% rate for the entire cohort. Further stratification by BMI showed that those with a BMI less than 30 had a significantly higher success rate (88.2%) compared with those with a BMI score between 30 and 40 (31.3%) and those with a BMI greater than 40 (16.7%). Hoff and colleagues[5] also confirmed the importance of BMI in determining surgical success for TORS base-of-tongue reduction, finding that those who were normal weight or overweight (BMI<30) had a significantly higher success rate compared with those who were obese (BMI>30).[16] The safety of this approach is reasonable because the main complication (bleeding) affected 4.2% of patients (range, 4.2%–5.3%). However, transient dysphagia (7.2%; range, 5%–14%) does compromise the quality of life and must be discussed with patients preoperatively. In a retrospective study, Eesa and colleagues[22] evaluated the short-term and long-term swallowing outcomes following TORS for OSAHS. In the short term (1 month postoperatively), there was minimal significant impact on the swallowing function (P = .56) based on the MD Anderson Dysphagia Inventory questionnaire. The degree of dysphagia was not correlated with the volume of tissue removed from the base of tongue, as shown by video fluoroscopic swallow study (VFSS) (P = .72). There were no complaints of swallowing dysfunction in the long term (up to 32 months postoperatively), and any complaints spontaneously resolved within 3 months postoperatively in all patients with initial abnormal findings on VFSS.[21]

Summary

OSAHS affects 2% to 4% of the adult population. This patient population tends to be morbidly obese with decreased lung and cardiovascular function. As a consequence, these patients are considered at greater risk of complications after surgery in general and of obstructive sleep apnea specifically.[15] OSAHS may increase rates of morbidity and mortality from numerous causes, such as increased blood pressure, insulin resistance, systemic inflammation, visceral fat deposition, and dyslipidemia, as well as cardiovascular disease, cerebrovascular disease, and metabolic syndrome. The increase in mortality from cardiovascular risk factors for patients with sleep apnea is in the moderate to severe range. If surgery reduces moderate or severe sleep apnea to mild sleep apnea, although not a cure, it is likely to significantly reduce the patient's neurocognitive and cardiopulmonary risk factors.

Obstruction in the retrolingual space can have several causes, including macroglossia, epiglottic prolapse, and lingual tonsil hypertrophy. Although TORS for OSAHS primarily addresses tongue base and supraglottic obstruction, it allows surgeons to address these obstructions with excellent visualization and a minimally invasive approach that is well tolerated by patients. TORS surgery supports 3 to 4 hands, whereas no more than 3 hands could be used in other traditional approaches. Moreover, the resection of a measurable portion of tongue seems to be another advantage of TORS surgery. It allows a wider surgical view and a more consistent removal of lingual tissue. In addition, the operating time is considerably less (30–90 minutes compared with several hours for non-robotic surgery). This point is critically important for patients with OSAHS, in whom extra soft tissue edema from prolonged retraction may significantly impede postoperative airway safety.[5]

The results demonstrate that TORS for base-of-tongue reduction successfully decreases AHI in most patients with OSAHS, as well as improving multiple sleep outcome measures. including LSAT, Epworth Sleepiness Scale, and snoring visual analog scales. The advantages described for TORS for base-of-tongue resection and lingual tonsillectomy compared with non-TORS methods of tongue reduction are reported to be improvement in magnification and surgical precision, avoidance of critical vessels and nerves, hemostatic control, and precise handling of tissues.[13] The application of TORS to the surgical treatment of OSAHS is still in its infancy; however, the results, so far, are promising, with early studies showing both safety and efficacy. By means of multiplanar tissue transection, at any angle it enhances the ability of surgeons in managing this complex region and, with respect to traditional open approaches, robotic management of the tongue base seems to be very well tolerated.[17]

References

1. Miller SC, Nguyen SA, Ong AA, et al. Transoral robotic base of tongue reduction for obstructive sleep apnea: a systematic review and meta-analysis. Laryngoscope 2017;127(1):258–65.
2. Lin HC, Hwang MS, Liao CC, et al. Taste disturbance following tongue base resection for OSA. Laryngoscope 2016;126(4):1009–13.
3. Arora A, Chaidas K, Garas G, et al. Outcome of TORS to tongue base and epiglottis in patients with OSA intolerant of conventional treatment. Sleep Breath 2016;20(2):739–47.
4. Lin HS, Rowley JA, Badr MS, et al. Transoral robotic surgery for treatment of obstructive sleep apnea-hypopnea syndrome. Laryngoscope 2013;123(7):1811–6.
5. Hoff PT, D'Agostino MA, Thaler ER. Transoral robotic surgery in benign diseases including obstructive sleep apnea: safety and feasibility. Laryngoscope 2015;125(5):1249–53.
6. D'Agostino MA. Transoral robotic partial glossectomy and supraglottoplasty for obstructive sleep apnea. Otolaryngol Clin North Am 2016;49(6):1415–23.
7. Vicini C, Montevecchi F, Gobbi R, et al. Transoral robotic surgery for obstructive sleep apnea syndrome: principles and technique. World J Otorhinolaryngol Head Neck Surg 2017;3(2):97–100.
8. Crawford JA, Montevecchi F, Vicini C, et al. Transoral robotic sleep surgery: the obstructive sleep apnea-hypopnea syndrome. Otolaryngol Clin North Am 2014;47(3):397–406.
9. Friedman M, Hamilton C, Samuelson CG, et al. Transoral robotic glossectomy for the treatment of obstructive sleep apnea-hypopnea syndrome. Otolaryngol Head Neck Surg 2012;146(5):854–62.
10. Vicini C, Montevecchi F, Campanini A, et al. Clinical outcomes and complications associated with TORS for OSAHS: a benchmark for evaluating an emerging surgical technology in a targeted application for benign disease. ORL J Otorhinolaryngol Relat Spec 2014; 76(2):63–9.
11. Hwang CS, Kim JW, Park SC, et al. Predictors of success in combination of tongue base resection and lateral pharyngoplasty for obstructive sleep apnea. Eur Arch Otorhinolaryngol 2017;274(5):2197–203.
12. Li S, Shi H. Lingual artery CTA-guided midline partial glossectomy for treatment of obstructive sleep apnea hypopnea syndrome. Acta Otolaryngol 2013;133(7):749–54.
13. Vicini C, Dallan I, Canzi P, et al. Transoral robotic surgery of the tongue base in obstructive sleep apnea-hypopnea syndrome: anatomic considerations and clinical experience. Head Neck 2012; 34(1):15–22.
14. Muderris T, Sevil E, Bercin S, et al. Transoral robotic lingual tonsillectomy in adults: preliminary results. Acta Otolaryngol 2015; 135(1):64–9.
15. Cillo JE Jr, Dattilo DJ. Early major medical complications after surgical management of obstructive sleep apnea: a retrospective cohort analysis and case series. J Oral Maxillofac Surg 2015;73(1): 123–8.
16. Glazer TA, Hoff PT, Spector ME. Transoral robotic surgery for obstructive sleep apnea: perioperative management and postoperative complications. JAMA Otolaryngol Head Neck Surg 2014; 140(12):1207–12.
17. Justin GA, Chang ET, Camacho M, et al. Transoral robotic surgery of obstructive sleep apnea: a systematic review and meta-analysis. Otolaryngol Head Neck Surg 2016;154(5):835–46.
18. Lin HS, Rowley JA, Folbe AJ, et al. Transoral robotic surgery for treatment of obstructive sleep apnea: factors predicting surgical response. Laryngoscope 2015;125(4):1013–20.
19. Richmon JD, Feng AL, Yang W, et al. Feasibility of rapid discharge after transoral robotic surgery of the oropharynx. Laryngoscope 2014;124(11):2518–25.
20. Koutsourelakis I, Safiruddin F, Ravesloot M, et al. Surgery for obstructive sleep apnea: sleep endoscopy determinants of outcome. Laryngoscope 2012;122(11):2587–91.
21. Meccariello G, Cammaroto G, Montevecchi F, et al. Transoral robotic surgery for the management of obstructive sleep apnea: a systematic review and meta-analysis. Eur Arch Otorhinolaryngol 2017;274(2):647–53.
22. Eesa M, Montevecchi F, Hendawy E, et al. Swallowing outcome after TORS for sleep apnea: short- and long-term evaluation. Eur Arch Otorhinolaryngol 2015;272(6):1537–41.

Pediatric Sleep Surgery

Skeletal Procedures

Cory M. Resnick, DMD, MD

KEYWORDS

• Obstructive sleep apnea • Robin sequence • Pierre robin sequence • Craniosynostosis • Syndromic craniosynostosis • Distraction osteogenesis

KEY POINTS

- Congenital craniofacial abnormalities are rare but often correctable causes of obstructive sleep apnea.
- Robin sequence and syndromic craniosynostosis are the most common congenital craniofacial anomalies associated with obstructive sleep apnea.
- Mandibular distraction is effective in relieving obstructive sleep apnea in properly selected patients with Robin sequence.
- Le Fort III midfacial distraction is effective in relieving obstructive sleep apnea in properly selected patients with syndromic craniosynostosis.

Video content accompanies this article at http://www.oralmaxsurgeryatlas.theclinics.com.

Introduction

Skeletal abnormalities are rare but often correctable causes of pediatric obstructive sleep apnea (OSA). Any facial abnormality that leads to airway impingement may contribute to OSA. The most common congenital craniofacial diagnoses associated with OSA are Robin sequence and syndromic craniosynostosis (SCS).

Robin sequence

Robin sequence (RS) is defined as the triad of micrognathia (small and retropositioned mandible), glossoptosis (tongue positioned superiorly and posteriorly such that it occludes the oropharynx), and airway obstruction. The incidence of RS ranges from 1:8500 to 1:14,000 live births. Although not a defining characteristic of RS, a cleft of the secondary palate is present in more than 90% of affected individuals.

The term "sequence" is applied to acknowledge a developmental progression beginning with micrognathia, which results in glossoptosis due to insufficient space in the oral cavity for normal tongue positioning (Fig. 1). The malpositioned tongue, in turn, obstructs the oropharynx and may inhibit fusion of the palatal shelves creating a U- or V-shaped cleft (Fig. 2). RS is not itself a syndrome; the initiating mandibular deformity can be attributed to one of more than 40 syndromic diagnoses or may be due to other extrinsic or intrinsic factors. Stickler and 22q11.2 syndromes are the most common syndromes associated with RS.

RS typically presents as airway obstruction and feeding impairment in the first few weeks of life. Some present later with failure to thrive. The airway obstruction associated with RS can often be managed with nonoperative maneuvers, including side or prone positioning, insertion of a nasopharyngeal tube or oral appliance, or continuous positive airway pressure. Many will experience mandibular catch-up growth and spontaneous resolution of the airway obstruction over the first year of life.

In infants with persistent obstruction despite nonoperative therapies, an operation is necessary. Tracheostomy is the most efficacious procedure, but is associated with significant morbidity, mortality, and social burden. Tongue-lip adhesion (TLA), which secures the anterior ventral tongue to the lower lip, thereby advancing the tongue base away from the oropharynx, is an alternative. Reported success rates range from 33% to 100%. In a 2015 analysis of TLA outcomes using polysomnographic data, Resnick and colleagues found that TLA improves but does not predictably resolve airway obstruction in patients with RS.

Mandibular distraction osteogenesis (MDO), which lengthens the mandible and brings the tongue forward, has gained popularity in treatment of infants with RS over the last decade. Compared with TLA, MDO more predictably improves breathing and avoids the need for tracheostomy in patients with RS. Success rates for MDO are 82% to 100%. Oral feeding has also been found to improve after MDO.

Surgical technique: mandibular distraction osteogenesis

Preoperative planning

The diagnosis and management of RS require a coordinated team approach, including expertise from neonatology,

Disclosure: The author has nothing to disclose.

Department of Plastic and Oral Surgery, Boston Children's Hospital, Harvard School of Dental Medicine, Harvard Medical School, 300 Longwood Avenue, Boston, MA 02115, USA

E-mail address: Cory.Resnick@childrens.harvard.edu

Atlas Oral Maxillofacial Surg Clin N Am 27 (2019) 67–75
1061-3315/19/
https://doi.org/10.1016/j.cxom.2018.11.001

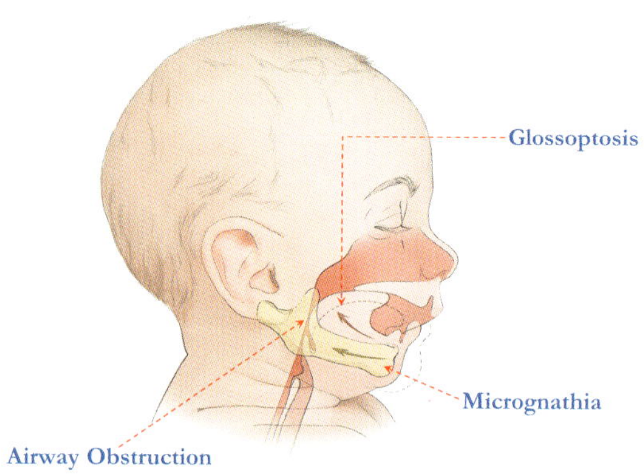

Fig. 1 The defining features of RS: micrognathia, glossoptosis, and airway obstruction.

genetics, pulmonology, gastroenterology, oral and maxillofacial surgery, otolaryngology, plastic surgery, anesthesia, and additional consultants as necessary. As clinical examination and continuous pulse oximetry underestimate the true incidence of OSA in infants, formal polysomnography is necessary to determine the severity of the apnea and rule out central apnea as a significant contributor to the respiratory distress.

Before an operation, it is critical to determine the site of airway obstruction. Bedside laryngoscopy may be used to assess the upper airway and vocal folds. Direct laryngoscopy and bronchoscopy, typically under general anesthesia, are necessary to evaluate subglottic structures.

If MDO is pursued, the operation can commence with or without preoperative virtual surgical planning (VSP) (Fig. 3). VSP allows for the fabrication of 3-dimensionally printed cutting guides and stereolithographic models (Fig. 4), aids in distraction device selection and placement, improves vector management, shortens and simplifies the operation, and may decrease injury to the inferior alveolar nerve and developing teeth.

Preparation and patient positioning

Careful perioperative airway management and preparation for a potentially difficult intubation are critical. A bronchoscopy and laryngoscopy are often performed at the beginning of the procedure, and intubation can be facilitated by the use of specialty equipment, such as an anterior commissure laryngoscope or an intubating fiberscope. Intubation can be from a nasal or oral approach; the curvature of a nasoendotracheal tube may improve stability of the tube and decrease the likelihood of accidental intraoperative extubation compared with an oroendoctracheal tube. The endoctracheal tube can be prepared in the sterile field, and the breathing circuit can be draped with a clear sterile ultrasound probe cover so that it is accessible for inspection and manipulation during the procedure. The entire face and neck are then prepared and draped.

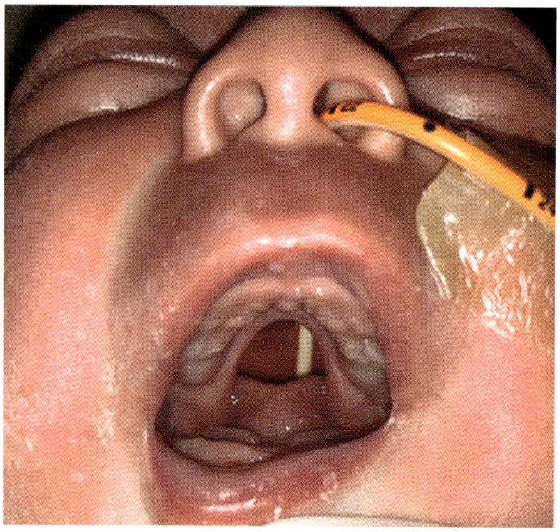

Fig. 2 A wide U-shaped cleft of the secondary palate in an infant with RS. A nasogastric tube enters the nose and is seen in the nasopharynx through the cleft palate.

Surgical procedure

The mandible is accessed via a 1-cm incision within a natural skin tension line 1 to 2 cm inferior to the mandibular inferior border (Video 1). Layered dissection is performed with identification and protection of the marginal mandibular nerve and management of the facial vessels as necessary. The mandibular angle and ramus are exposed, and the cutting guides are used, when available from preoperative VSP, to mark the planned osteotomies and device positions.

The goals in osteotomy design are to (1) minimize or avoid damage to developing teeth and the inferior alveolar nerve, (2) avoid binding of the mobilized distal segment against the proximal segment during distraction, (3) avoid bringing the coronoid process forward with the distal segment, because this could lead to impingement with the zygomatic arch during distraction, (4) provide sufficient bone in each segment for device fixation, (5) achieve the desired vector for distraction, and (6) match the distraction vector between sides. Based on these criteria, the osteotomy can be custom designed for each patient. Common osteotomy designs include linear oblique, inverted-L, and multiangular (Fig. 5). The osteotomy is created with a piezo electric saw, with only a buccal corticotomy in the midportion over the inferior alveolar nerve. This technique avoids damage to the nerve and maintains continuity of the mandible for stability while the device is applied.

Either a buried internal device (Fig. 6) or an external distraction device with percutaneous pins can be used. When using an internal device, the device is applied with at least 4 screws in each footplate. The turning mechanism can extend either posteriorly and emerge under the lobule of the ear (Fig. 7) or anteriorly to emerge inferior the mandibular body. After application of the device, the osteotomy is completed at the remaining lingual plate with an osteotome. The operation is repeated on the contralateral side. The device is activated 1.5 to 2 mm, and the segments are observed for complete separation without tension. The wound is closed in layers, and the operation is repeated on the contralateral side.

Immediate postoperative care

Patients often remain intubated for 2 to 3 days postoperatively to allow for resolution of airway swelling that results from intubation and fluid shifts associated with the operation. A short latency period may be used, after which distraction commences at a rate of 1 to 3 mm per day. At Boston Children's Hospital, distraction begins on the first postoperative day with 2 mm of advancement on that day and each day thereafter, separated into morning and afternoon turns. The most common end-distraction target is when the mandibular alveolar ridge is 2 to 4 mm anterior to the maxillary alveolar ridge. Once active distraction has completed, the turning arms are removed at the bedside. The average advancement is 20 mm (Fig. 8).

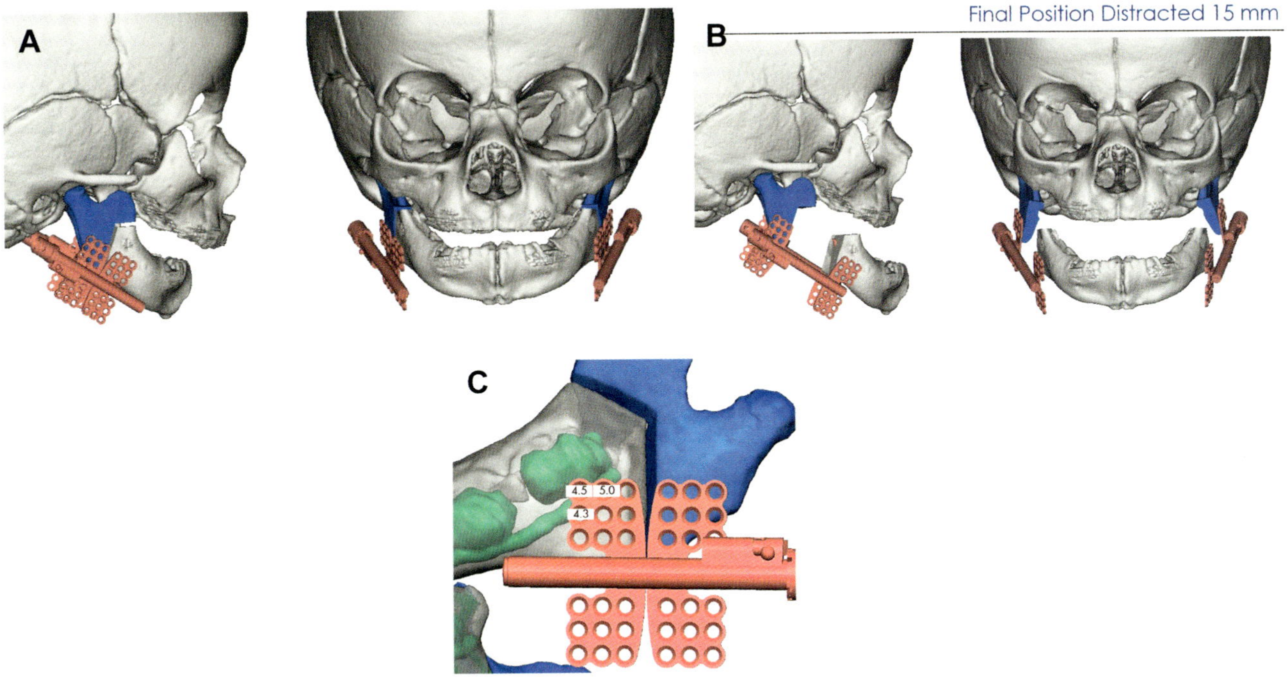

Fig. 3 VSP for mandibular distraction in an infant with RS. (*A*) Planned osteotomy and position of distraction device. (*B*) Simulated distraction. (*C*) Relationship of planned distractor position to developing teeth and the inferior alveolar nerve. The distance from the buccal cortex to these underlying structures is shown in millimeters and is helpful in planning the osteotomy and positions for fixation screws.

Patients may be discharged home either during the distraction process, if appropriate, or immediately after removal of the activation arms, unless comorbidities require continued hospitalization. At Boston Children's Hospital, a polysomnogram is repeated to confirm the resolution of OSA before discharge. Devices are removed after a 6- to 12-week consolidation period.

Potential complications

There are many opportunities for error in the surgical management of the infant with RS with MDO. These errors include the following:

- Incorrect/incomplete diagnosis. Appropriate surgical management begins with an accurate diagnosis and workup. If comorbidities that contribute to respiratory distress, such as hypotonia or central apnea, are not recognized and managed, mandibular distraction may fail to relieve the OSA.
- Nonrecognition of concomitant airway lesions. Similar to incomplete diagnosis, failure to address other contributing airway lesions, including laryngomalacia, may lead to an unsatisfactory outcome.
- Airway mismanagement. Intubation may be difficult in the patient with RS and requires special expertise and equipment.
- Incomplete osteotomy. If the mandibular osteotomy is incomplete, the segments will not move as expected and the distraction process will halt prematurely. It is imperative to evaluate all areas of the osteotomy and test the mobility of the segments intraoperatively.
- Damage to teeth and nerves. Developing teeth and the inferior alveolar nerve are at risk during the mandibular osteotomy. This risk may be minimized with VSP. The marginal mandibular branch of the facial nerve must also be recognized and protected during the dissection.
- Device detachment. The bone of the mandible may be narrow and poorly calcified, particularly in neonates.

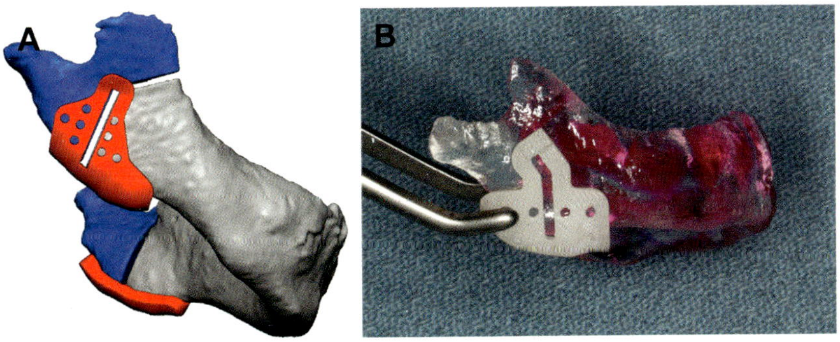

Fig. 4 (*A*) Cutting guides are designed based on the virtual surgical plan. (*B*) The cutting guides can be used with a 3-dimensionally printed mandibular model to prebend distraction devices and plan the operation.

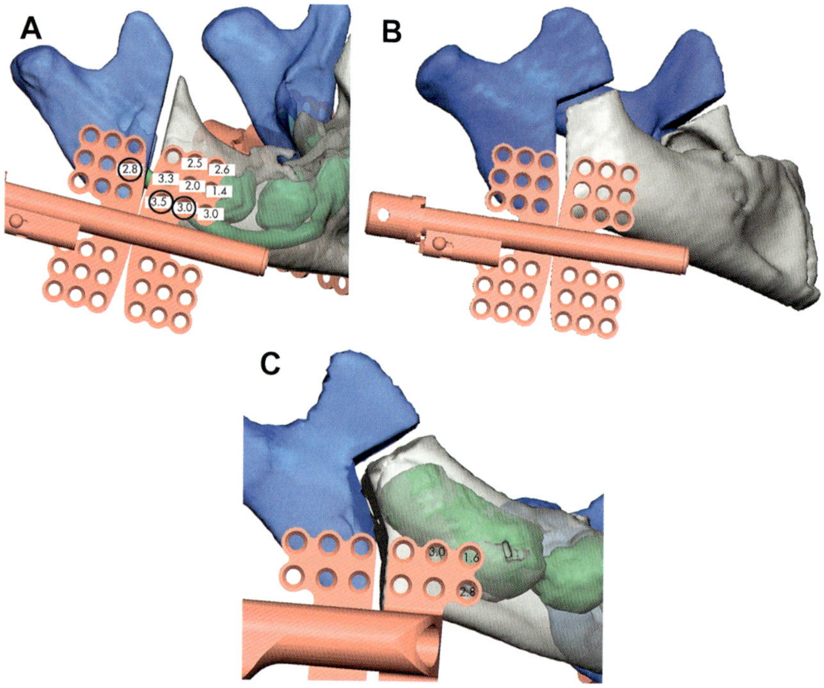

Fig. 5 Common osteotomy designs for infant mandibular distraction: (*A*) linear oblique, (*B*) inverted L, (*C*) multiangular. (*From* Resnick CM. Precise osteotomies for mandibular distraction in infants with Robin sequence using virtual surgical planning. Int J Oral Maxillofac Surg 2018;47(1):35–43; with permission.)

Careful application of bone screws and assessment of the device stability intraoperatively are important to minimize the risk of device detachment during distraction or consolidation.

- Device malfunction. The distraction device may fail to operate properly during the distraction or consolidation phases, or components may break. This may require additional operations to repair or exchange devices, particularly when internal devices are used.
- Pin scars. When external devices are used, unsightly pin scars may result from movement of the percutaneous pins through the skin during distraction.
- Infection. Subcutaneous infections, particularly at the site of emergence of the distractor activation mechanism when internal devices are used, are common. Diligent wound care is crucial, and perioperative antibiotics are often necessary. Infection may occasionally dictate early removal of distraction devices. Osteomyelitis is exceedingly rare.
- Nonunion. A nonunion can occur if bone consolidation within the distraction gaps and fusion of the proximal and distal mandibular segments are inhibited. This can occur if the distraction rate is too fast, if a comorbidity decreases bone turnover, or may be idiopathic.
- Premature consolidation. An inadequate rate of distraction may lead to premature consolidation. This may necessitate a repeat operation.
- Disruption of future growth. The effect of distraction on future mandibular growth is unknown. Some patients will require repeated distraction; this may be due to disruption of growth by the first procedure or an inherent mandibular growth abnormality.

"Pearls and pitfalls"

Experience with patients with RS has led to improvement in management. Recommendations based on this experience include the following:

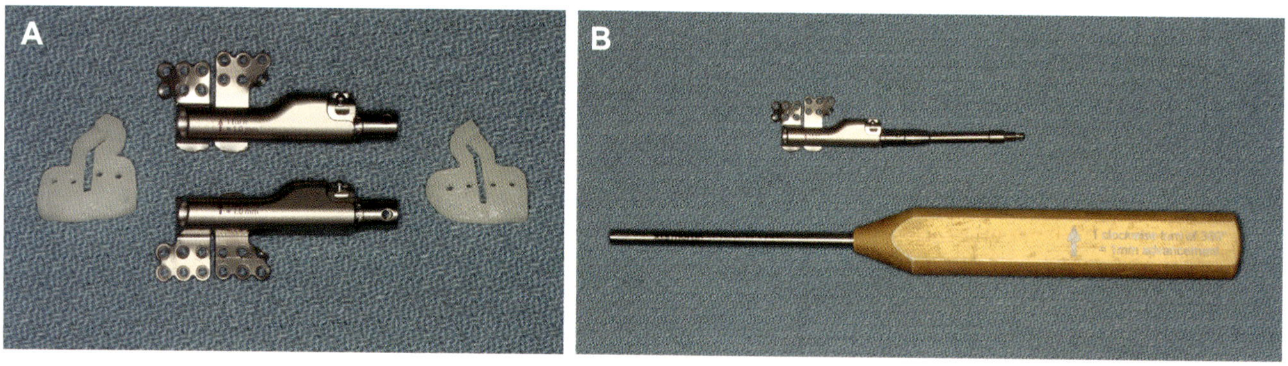

Fig. 6 Buried internal distraction device. (*A*) Prebent devices and cutting guides. (*B*) Device with detachable turning mechanism and turning driver.

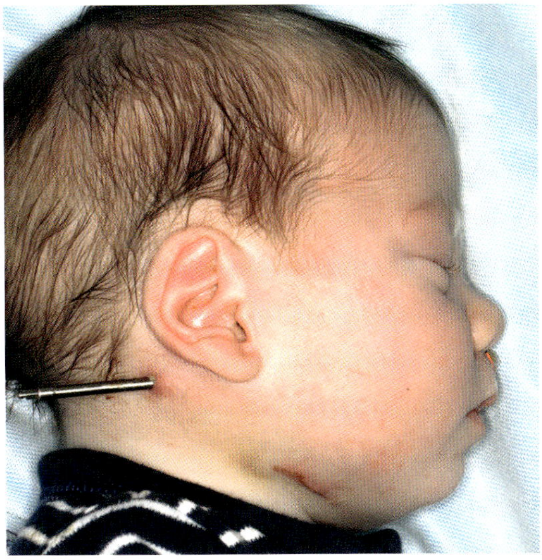

Fig. 7 Turning mechanism emerging posteriorly under the ear lobule. (*From* Resnick CM. Precise osteotomies for mandibular distraction in infants with Robin sequence using virtual surgical planning. Int J Oral Maxillofac Surg 2018;47(1):35–43; with permission.)

- Always perform a direct laryngoscopy and bronchoscopy before pursuing mandibular distraction or any other operation intended to relieve airway obstruction. Lack of recognition of concomitant airway lesions may lead to an operative failure.
- Preoperative polysomnography, when available, may help in determining the best management plan. The presence and degree of obstruction cannot be adequately evaluated by bedside examination and monitoring.
- Engage in preoperative discussion with the anesthesia provider, with particular focus on the following:
  - Airway management plan
  - Expected and allowable blood loss
  - Avoidance of neuromuscular blockade to facilitate monitoring for the marginal mandibular nerve
- During the preparation and drape, apply a clear sterile ultrasound probe cover over the endotracheal tube and breathing circuit to allow them to be visualized during the procedure. The ability of team members to visualize and manipulate the endotracheal tube and breathing circuit throughout the case has reduced accidental intraoperative extubation, particularly during head turns.
- When planning the mandibular osteotomy, leave sufficient proximal bone for device application. Placement of the osteotomy proximal to the mandibular canal is ideal for protection of the inferior alveolar nerve and may be achievable in older children, but is usually impossible in infants. The osteotomy typically overlaps the inferior alveolar nerve canal in younger patients to provide adequate proximal bone for device fixation.
- When the osteotomy overlaps the inferior alveolar nerve canal, the nerve can be preserved by identifying its location on preoperative imaging and performing only a buccal corticotomy over this area with a piezo electric saw. The separation of the proximal and distal segments is completed later by driving an osteotome along the lingual cortex. Using this technique, the nerve is typically seen within the osteotomy gap (Fig. 9) and will elongate during the distraction process.
- Tactile sensation of proper device positioning can be aided by prebending the most posterior-inferior screw hole to wrap around the mandibular angle. When the device is inserted, a catch will be felt when this screw hole is positioned as planned.
- Confirm intraoperatively that the osteotomy is complete, the proximal and distal segments separate passively, and the distraction device functions properly.
- Attempt to match the distraction vector between the left and ride side and avoid overconvergence of device paths. Mismatched vectors and overconvergence create undue pressure on the devices and the mandibular condyles and may lead to device failure and/or condylar dysfunction.

Syndromic craniosynostosis

Craniosynostosis, the premature fusion of one or more sutures of the cranial vault, leads to growth restriction perpendicular to the fused suture or sutures and compensatory growth in the other sutures. Most craniosynostoses are nonsyndromic. SCS occurs in 1:25,000 to 1:100,000 of live births and typically

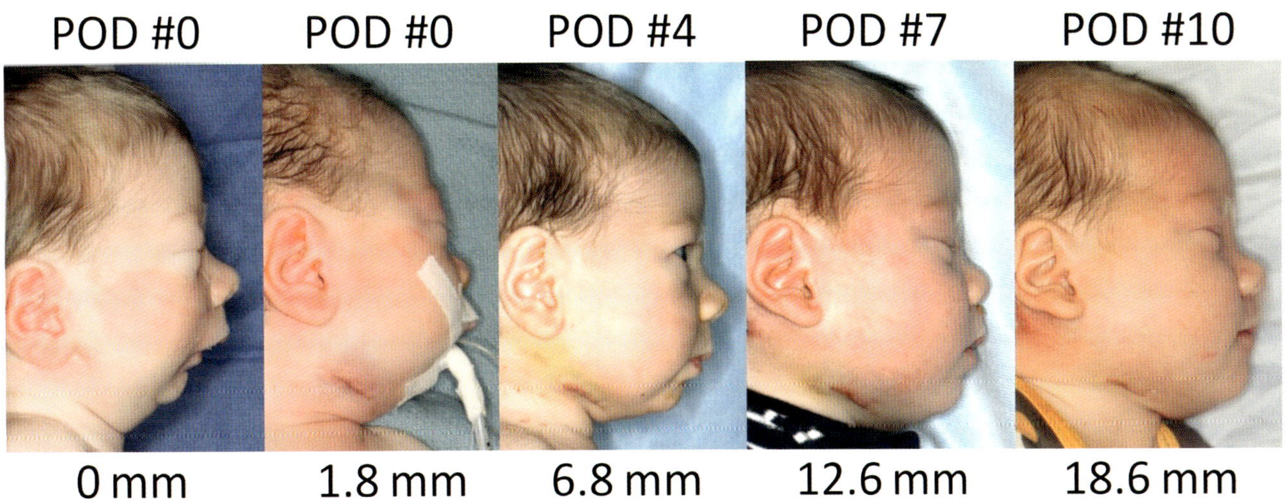

Fig. 8 Sequential advancement of the mandible from postoperative day (POD) #0 to POD #10 during the active phase of mandibular distraction.

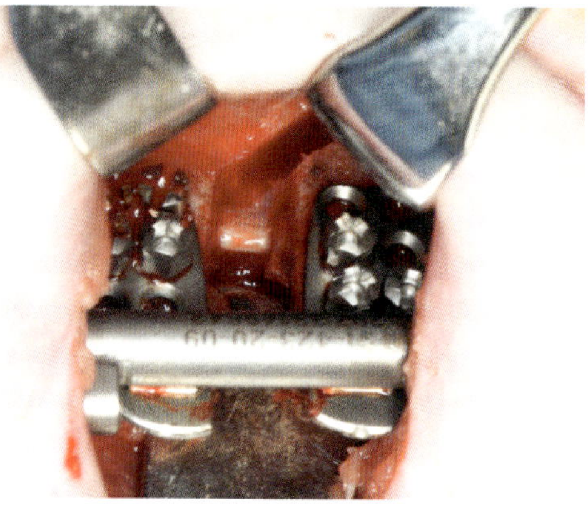

Fig. 9 The inferior alveolar nerve is preserved during the mandibular osteotomy and is seen within the distraction gap when the device is tested intraoperatively.

involves multiple cranial sutures. Any involved suture pattern is possible; turribrachycephaly due to synostotic bilateral coronal, frontosphenoidal, and sphenoethmoidal sutures is most common. Some SCS have additional extracraniofacial features such as hand and feet anomalies. Fibroblast growth factor receptor genes have been implicated in some SCS.

Midfacial retrusion is a hallmark of some SCS, particularly Apert, Crouzon, and Pfeiffer syndromes. This midfacial hypoplasia results in exorbitism (Fig. 10), malocclusion, and narrowing of the nasopharyngeal airway. Inverso and colleagues demonstrated that more than half of patients with SCS have symptoms of OSA, and, of those, two-thirds have confirmed OSA by polysomnography. The OSA is severe in at least one-fourth.

Patients with SCS typically require several skeletal operations during childhood. Key considerations in the need and timing for these operations include the following:

- Intracranial hypertension (ICH). ICH will be present in at least 50% of patients with SCS, and, if uncorrected, can result in poor neurodevelopment and Chiari malformation (herniation of the hindbrain). Signs of ICH include bulging of the fontanelles, cranial suture diastasis, papilledema, "thumb printing" of the skull, ventriculomegaly, and failure to thrive. The presence of ICH may necessitate an operation to increase cranial volume.
- Ocular protection. Many patients with SCS have exorbitism and proptosis due to retruded supraorbital and infraorbital rims and small bony orbits (see Fig. 10). This creates a risk for exposure keratitis and ulceration. Because the orbital rims provide inadequate globe protection, some patients will experience eye injury and even blindness from minor trauma. Optic nerve atrophy can also occur from uncorrected ICH.
- OSA. The severity of the OSA response to nonoperative maneuvers may dictate timing for skeletal surgery. In those patients with tracheostomies, decannulation may be a goal of surgery. Nelson and colleagues demonstrated that midfacial distraction leads to significant improvement of OSA in patients with SCS.
- Psychosocial development. Visible facial differences are associated with impaired social development and psychiatric disease. Surgical improvement of the facial deformity has been shown to lead to improved psychosocial well-being.

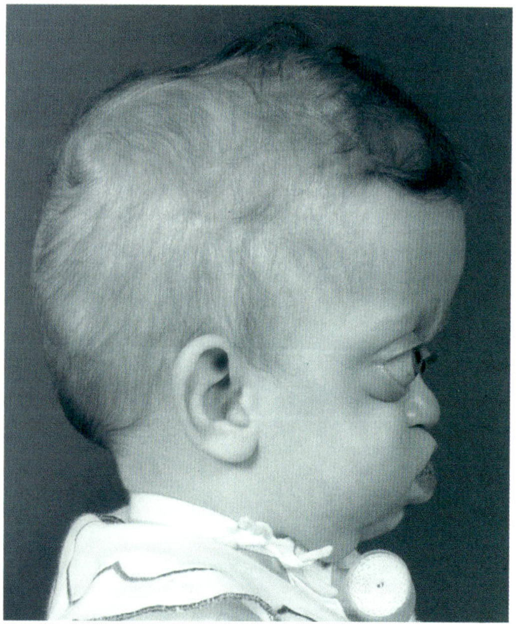

Fig. 10 Patient with Pfeiffer syndrome, severe midfacial hypoplasia, exorbitism, and proptosis.

Surgical technique: Le Fort III midfacial advancement

Preoperative planning

As for RS, the diagnosis and management of SCS necessitate a coordinated team and is often relegated to large craniofacial centers. Careful consideration should be given to the staging of skeletal operations. As bone growth may be diminished postoperatively, delaying an operation until the skeletal structures at risk have matured is best, unless other considerations indicate earlier operation. Midfacial structures reach adult proportions by around the age of 12 years; this is an ideal time to proceed with Le Fort III midfacial advancement. The presence of severe OSA and/or a drive to decannulate a tracheostomy are common indications for Le Fort III midfacial advancement during growth (Fig. 11). When pursuing this operation during growth, the patient and family should be informed of the potential need to repeat the midfacial advancement after skeletal maturity.

A computed tomography scan that includes the skull and maxillofacial structures should be obtained before Le Fort III osteotomy. VSP and 3-dimensional printing of cutting guides can be used to identify ideal osteotomies and aid placement of distraction devices, particularly when internal distractors are used. Printing of a stereolithographic model of the skull and face is helpful in visualizing the 3-dimensional facial anatomy and prebending device foot plates.

Preparation and patient positioning

After the induction of anesthesia, the patient is intubated orally. The endotracheal tube can be secured using a circumdental or circummandibular wire. The hair is shaved as necessary and tied in bunches. Lubricant is applied to the eyes, and tarsorrhaphy sutures are placed in the lids. The entire head and neck are then prepared in to the sterile field. Tumescent solution can be placed in the scalp for hemostasis and hydrodissection.

Surgical procedure

The oral clean-contaminated portion of the procedure is performed first. After infiltration with local anesthetic containing

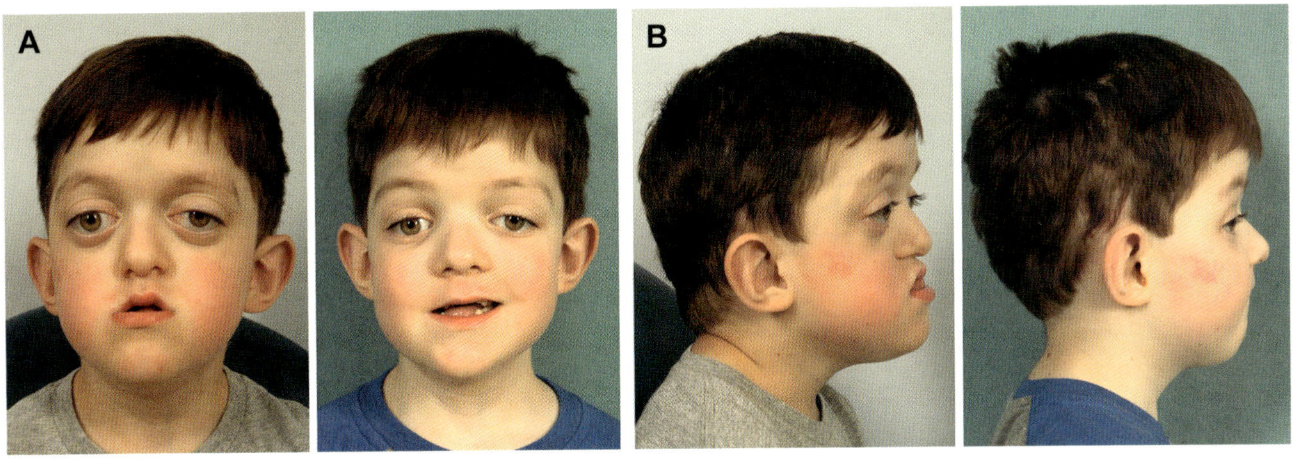

Fig. 11 Patient with Crouzon syndrome who had Le Fort III midfacial distraction at age 6 years for severe OSA. The OSA completely resolved postoperatively. Before and after frontal (*A*) and lateral (*B*) photographs.

vasoconstrictor, an incision is created in the maxillary buccal vestibule on each side. A subperiosteal flap is elevated to access the infraorbital rims and pterygomaxillary junctions on each side, while preserving the infraorbital nerves. Elevating the periosteum of the infraorbital rims, some of the lateral orbital rims and the anterior orbital floors from the transoral approach will facilitate connection of the oral dissection with the coronal approach that follows. A long curved osteotome is used to separate the posterior maxilla from the pterygoid plates on each side. If an external halo distractor with internal footplates is to be used, the footplates can be secured to the maxillary buttresses at this time. Transoral access for foot plate application may necessitate skeletonizing the infraorbital nerves and/or osteotomizing the bone superior to the infraorbital foramina to allow the nerves to move into the orbits.

Preparation and drape are then repeated for the sterile portion of the procedure. A coronal incision is made within the hairline, and dissection to the supraorbital rims is performed in either a subgaleal or a subpericranial plane. If the patient has previously had a cranioplasty and/or long-standing ICH, special care must be taken to avoid entering holes in the skull and puncturing the dura during this dissection. Preoperative imaging can be used to identify the location of these danger areas. Dissection is continued in a subpericranial/subperiosteal plane onto the nasal bones, around the orbital rims, and onto the zygomatic arches. The dissection plane is connected at the orbital rims to the transoral wounds.

An osteotomy is made with a reciprocating or piezo electric saw at the zygomaticotemporal sutures on each side. The saw is then used to osteotomize the lateral orbits from the inferior orbital fissures to the frontozygomatic sutures. The next osteotomy is at the nasofrontal suture, extending slightly onto the medial orbital walls. The medial and lateral orbital osteotomies are connected along the soft bone of the orbital floor behind the infraorbital rim, the medial orbit, and lamina papyracea behind the lacrimal apparatus with a sharp

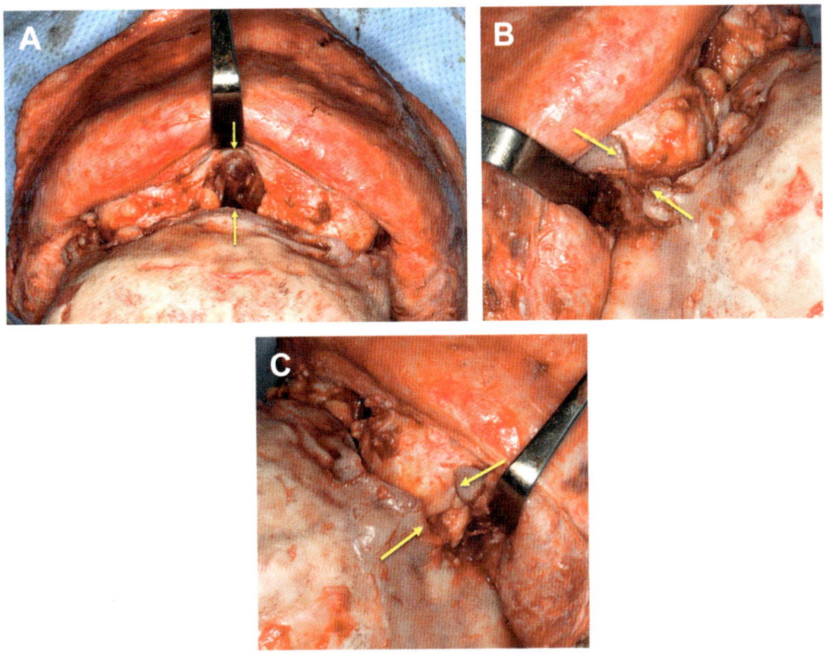

Fig. 12 Separation with minimal tension should be observed at the nasofrontal suture (*A*) and bilateral zygomaticofrontal sutures (*B*, *C*). Gaps between osseous segments are indicated by yellow arrows.

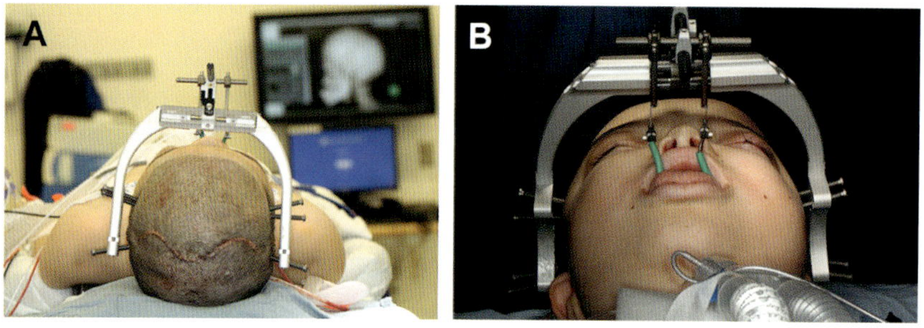

Fig. 13 External halo midfacial distraction device viewed from above (*A*) and below (*B*).

instrument such as a diamond blade or periosteal elevator. A long curved osteotome is then used to osteotomize the bony nasal septum from the nasofrontal suture to the posterior nasal spine. A finger is applied transorally to the posterior nasal spine to palpate the osteotome as it reaches this position. The pterygoid osteotomies that were started from the transoral approach are then completed with the long curved osteotome from the coronal wound.

The midface is gently mobilized with osteotomes, pterygoid lifts, and Rowe disimpaction forceps. All osteotomies are carefully observed during mobilization to ensure that they are complete (Fig. 12). If significant resistance to mobilization is encountered, the osteotomies are refined until mobilization with minimal tension is achieved.

If intraoperative repositioning and fixation of the midface are planned, the occlusal splint and intermaxillary fixation are applied to dictate the final midfacial position. Bone grafts are harvested and inserted, and rigid fixation is applied. If distraction osteogenesis is used, then the devices are applied at this time. If an external halo distraction device is used, then the internal components are inserted, and the halo is applied after wound closure (Fig. 13). The wounds are irrigated and closed in layers.

Immediate postoperative care

Patients remain intubated for 2 to 3 days postoperatively. The tarsorrhaphy sutures are maintained during the intubated period to decrease chemosis and are removed when extubation is imminent. A short latency period may be used, and distraction is performed at a rate of 1 to 3 mm per day. At Boston Children's Hospital, distraction commences on the second or third postoperative day, with 2 mm of advancement on that day and each day thereafter, separated into morning and afternoon turns.

Patients are typically discharged home during the distraction process, with visits every several days to monitor progress. The target endpoint for midfacial distraction is normalization of orbital-globe relationships, specifically with the infraorbital rims 2 to 3 mm anterior to the *apex corneae*. Distraction devices are removed after an 8- to 12-week consolidation period.

Potential complications

As with mandibular distraction in RS, there are several potential complications with Le Fort III midfacial distraction. Many of these are similar to those described for RS and mandibular distraction in earlier discussion. Additional possible complications include the following:

- Dural tear. In patients with SCS who have had long-standing ICH and prior cranioplasties, there are often persistent holes and weaknesses in the frontal bone. Care must be taken during the coronal dissection to avoid penetrating the dura in these areas and causing leakage of cerebrospinal fluid.
- Globe injury and blindness. The eyes and orbital nerves must be carefully protected during the Le Fort III osteotomy. Corneal abrasion or more severe globe injury, possibly leading to blindness, can occur.
- Fracture of the maxilla/midface. During mobilization of the midface, fractures, particularly at the zygomas or in the midline of the palate, may occur. This can be prevented by ensuring that all osteotomies are complete before mobilization and by pushing forward from behind the maxilla rather than pulling from the front as the initial method for mobilization (see Fig. 12).
- Disruption of future growth. As for the mandible in RS, there may be a growth inhibitory effect to Le Fort III osteotomy before skeletal maturity. When indications for an earlier operation are not present, this operation should be delayed until skeletal maturity.

"Pearls and pitfalls"

Experience with the Le Fort III osteotomy has led to many observations and innovations. Some observations and innovations include the following:

- Customize the operation to the deformity. Many modifications are possible, such as excluding the nasal bones if the nasal bridge is prominent, segmenting the midface, and/or advancing the lateral portions of the midface more than the central portion.
- Use a 3-dimensionally printed stereolithographic model to evaluate the anatomy preoperatively. This is particularly helpful in identifying defects in the frontal bone that may be encountered during the dissection, determining the angle for the nasal septal separation to avoid damage to the cribiform plate, and in prebending distraction device foot plates.
- Carefully consider the vector of distraction when applying an external halo device. There is a tendency for the midface to rotate in a counterclockwise direction during distraction, which may result in an abnormal maxillary occlusal plane and anterior open bite. This can be compensated for by adjusting the device intraoperatively.
- Consider the Le Fort III osteotomy as one of several stages in correction of the SCS deformity. Although this operation may be used to correct both the orbital-globe relationships and the occlusal discrepancy, with or without a simultaneous Le Fort I osteotomy, attempting to accomplish too much during a single operation risks compromising the success of the procedure.

Summary

Skeletal operations may be effective in relieving OSA in patients with craniofacial deformities. RS, in which the oropharyngeal airway is obstructed by glossoptosis resulting from micrognathia, and SCS, in which the nasopharyngeal airway is impinged by midfacial hypoplasia, are 2 examples.

Supplementary data

Supplementary data related to this article can be found online at https://doi.org/10.1016/j.cxom.2018.11.001

Further readings

Almajed A, Viezel-Mathieu A, Gilardino MS, et al. Outcome following surgical nterventions for micrognathia in infants with pierre Robin sequence: a systematic review of the literature. Cleft Palate Craniofac J 2017;54(1):32–42.

Breik O, Tivey D, Umapathysivam K, et al. Does the rate of distraction or type of distractor affect the outcome of mandibular distraction in children with micrognathia? J Oral Maxillofac Surg 2016;74(7):1441–53.

Collins B, Powitzky R, Robledo C, et al. Airway management in pierre Robin sequence: patterns of practice. Cleft Palate Craniofac J 2014;51:283–9.

Evans KN, Sie KC, Hopper RA, et al. Robin sequence: from diagnosis to development of an effective management plan. Pediatrics 2011; 127(5):936–48.

Hollier LH Jr, Higuera S, Stal S, et al. Distraction rate and latency: factors in the outcome of pediatric mandibular distraction. Plast Reconstr Surg 2006;117(7):2333–6.

Hollier LH, Kim JH, Grayson B, et al. Mandibular growth after distraction in patients under 48 months of age. Plast Reconstr Surg 1999; 103(5):1361–70.

Hopper R, Kapadia H, Morton T. Normalizing facial ratios in apert syndrome patients with le fort II midface distraction and simultaneous zygomatic repositioning. Plast Reconstr Surg 2013;132(1):129–40.

Inverso G, Brustowicz KA, Katz E, et al. The prevalence of obstructive sleep apnea in symptomatic patients with syndromic craniosynostosis. Int J Oral Maxillofac Surg 2016;45(2):167–9.

Katz ES, Mitchell RB, D'Ambrosio CM. Obstructive sleep apnea in infants. Am J Respir Crit Care Med 2012;185(8):805–16.

Kolstad CK, Senders CW, Rubinstein BK, et al. Mandibular distraction osteogenesis: at what age to proceed. Int J Pediatr Otorhinolaryngol 2011;75(11):1380–4.

Nelson TE, Mulliken JB, Padwa BL. Effect of midfacial distraction on the obstructed airway in patients with syndromic bilateral coronal synostosis. J Oral Maxillofac Surg 2008;66(11):2318–21.

Paes EC, Mink van der Molen AB, Muradin MSM, et al. A systematic review on the outcome of mandibular distraction osteogenesis in infants suffering Robin sequence. Clin Oral Investig 2013;17(8): 1807–20.

Papoff P, Guelfi G, Cicchetti R, et al. Outcomes after tongue-lip adhesion or mandibular distraction osteogenesis in infants with Pierre Robin sequence and severe airway obstruction. Int J Oral Maxillofac Surg 2013;42(11):1418–23.

Resnick CM, Kooiman TD, Calabrese CE, et al. An algorithm for predicting Robin sequence from fetal MRI. Prenat Diagn 2018;38(5): 357–64.

Resnick CM, Dentino K, Katz E, et al. Effectiveness of tongue-lip adhesion for obstructive sleep apnea in infants with Robin sequence measured by polysomnography. Cleft Palate Craniofac J 2016;53(5): 584–8.

Resnick CM, Rottgers SA, Langenfeld CC, et al. Novel rigid external distraction device improves stability and controls the vector during midfacial advancement. J Craniofac Surg 2016;27(4): 1056–9.

Resnick CM. Precise osteotomies for mandibular distraction in infants with Robin sequence using virtual surgical planning. Int J Oral Maxillofac Surg 2018;47(1):35–43.

Scott AR, Tibesar RJ, Lander TA, et al. Mandibular distraction osteogenesis in infants younger than 3 months. Arch Facial Plast Surg 2011;13(3):173–9.

Steinberg JP, Brady CM, Waters BR, et al. Mid-term dental and nerve-related complications of infant distraction for Robin sequence. Plast Reconstr Surg 2016;138(1):82e–90e.

Tahiri Y, Viezel-Mathieu A, Aldekhayel S, et al. The effectiveness of mandibular distraction in improving airway obstruction in the pediatric population. Plast Reconstr Surg 2014;133(3):352e–9e.

Tibesar RJ, Scott AR, McNamara C, et al. Distraction osteogenesis of the mandible for airway obstruction in children: long-term results. Otolaryngol Head Neck Surg 2010;143(1):90–6.

Pediatric Tongue Base Surgery

Gi Soo Lee, MD, EdM [a,b], Umakanth Katwa, MD [c,d,*]

KEYWORDS

• Glossoptosis • Lingual tonsillectomy • Tongue base excision

KEY POINTS

- Tongue base is one of the most common sites of upper airway obstruction in patients with persistent obstructive sleep apnea after removal of adenoids and palatine tonsils.
- Tongue base obstruction can be caused by hypertrophied lingual tonsils (LT) and/or glossoptosis (retrograde collapse of tongue parenchyma).
- Obstruction of the tongue base should be confirmed with drug-induced sleep endoscopy (DISE) and or cine MRI of upper airways.
- Lingual tonsillar hypertrophy can be differentiated from glossoptosis by performing tongue extension (for LT hypertrophy) or jaw thrust maneuvers (for glossoptosis) during DISE.

Introduction: nature of the problem

Tongue base obstruction (TBO) is a common cause of persistent obstructive sleep apnea (OSA) after removal of adenoids and tonsils in children, particularly in those with rapid eye movement (REM) or supine-dominant OSA. The tongue is part of the collapsible pharyngeal airway and most amenable to collapse because of either loss of genioglossus tone during REM sleep or gravity-dependent collapse into the oropharyngeal airway during sleeping in the supine position. The tongue base, defined as the posterior one-third of the tongue from the circumvallate papillae to the vallecula, comprises both tongue musculature and the lingual tonsil (LT). The degree of TBO depends on 2 factors: LT hypertrophy and glossoptosis; sometimes both coexist. Obstruction of the laryngeal airway can be caused by either or both glossoptosis (retrograde collapse of the tongue) and LT hypertrophy. The most common risk factors for LT hypertrophy include Down syndrome, obesity, and significant allergies. In addition, children with Down syndrome have macroglossia and glossoptosis resulting in significant TBO.

Removal of LT and/or reduction in tongue base bulk can increase the retrolingual space and minimize the obstructive tendencies over the laryngeal inlet. Persistence of nasal obstruction may increase the negative pressure in the pharyngeal airway leading to worsening of the tongue base collapse; hence, it is critical to simultaneously assess and treat significant nasal obstruction.

Disclosure: The authors have nothing to disclose.

[a] Department of Otolaryngology and Communication Enhancement, Boston Children's Hospital, 300 Longwood Ave, Boston, MA 02115, USA
[b] Department of Otolaryngology, Harvard Medical School, 25 Shattuck St, Boston, MA 02115, USA
[c] Department of Pediatrics, Division of Pulmonary and Sleep Medicine, Boston Children's Hospital, 300 Longwood Ave, Boston, MA 02115, USA
[d] Department of Pediatrics, Harvard Medical School, 25 Shattuck St, Boston, MA 02115, USA
* Corresponding author. 27 Intervale Road, Chestnut Hill, MA 02467.
E-mail address: Umakanth.Katwa@childrens.harvard.edu

Diagnostic modalities

Polysomnography (sleep study)

TBO can present with snoring and obstructive sleep disordered breathing that is particularly worse in REM sleep and in the supine position. The sleep study helps to assess the severity of the upper airway obstruction. If the LTs are massive, obstructive events are evident in both REM and non–rapid eye movement (NREM) sleep. However, at times, markedly enlarged LTs can present with a milder degree of OSA if the genioglossus muscle is able to contract and maintain the tone during sleep without causing glossoptosis. It is critical to analyze the sleep study parameters in detail and assess the severity and the extent of OSA in REM and NREM sleep and in the supine position. Also, one should evaluate obstructive apnea index (OAI) and obstructive hypopnea index (OHI) separately. Successful treatment of TBO may result in a significant reduction in obstructive apneas (OAI). Sometimes, however, the persistent OSA after lingual tonsillectomy may show mostly hypopneic events rather than apneic obstructive events with a modest change in the overall combined obstructive apnea and hypopnea index (OAHI). These hypopneic events are particularly likely if the TBO is also associated with glossoptosis. Hence, a preoperative and a postoperative sleep study should be done in any patient being treated with tongue base surgery (Fig. 1).

Imaging studies

Imaging studies may include lateral neck films to assess air column in the retroglossal space and soft tissue shadow of LTs. However, plain films may not be accurate many times because it is typically done while awake and in the erect position. A

Atlas Oral Maxillofacial Surg Clin N Am 27 (2019) 77-81

https://doi.org/10.1016/j.cxom.2018.11.003

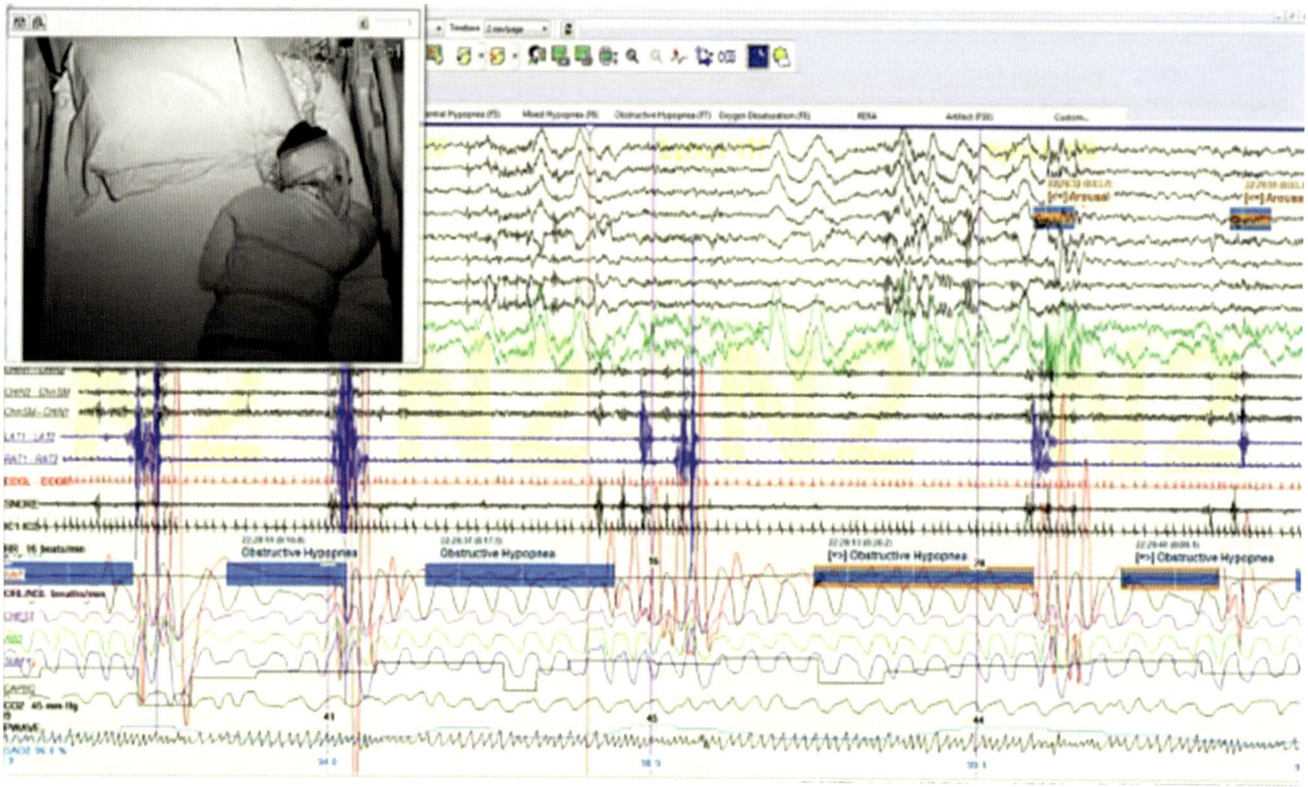

Fig. 1 A 2-minute sleep study epoch shows severe residual OSA (OAHI 65/h) with recurrent obstructive hypopneas in an 8-year-old boy who had undergone adenotonsillectomy for OSA. DISE revealed LT hypertrophy. LT removal led to complete resolution of OSA (OAHI 1/h).

cone beam computed tomography (CBCT) scan of the upper airway may be better in delineating the bony as well as soft tissue structures; in addition, one can measure the volume of the airways in the retroglossal area. Again, CBCT scans are done while awake and in the erect position and hence fail to assess glossoptosis seen during sleep. Cine MRI is a high-resolution imaging study that captures the dynamic movement of the upper airways during a medically induced sleeplike state. The major advantage of cine MRI over drug-induced sleep endoscopy (DISE) is that it can differentiate LT hypertrophy–related TBO from glossoptosis and help visualize the multilevel obstruction simultaneously.[1] This technique is not widely available and not used routinely. Sometimes cine MRI can be used as a complementary test to DISE.

Airway upper airway endoscopy

Awake flexible laryngoscopy can be done in clinic and help visualize airways from nose to larynx. Although it helps to visualize LTs, it cannot accurately assess glossoptosis seen during sleep; however, one can predict this based on the degree of laryngeal visualization. However, it is still a very useful tool. As DISE is performed in a medically induced sleeplike state like cine MRI, it is more effective in evaluating the site and the degree of TBO, and it most closely resembles events happening during sleep.[1–4] Various grading systems have been developed to assess the severity of glossoptosis (Yellon grading system for epiglottic and tongue-base prolapse) and lingual tonsillar hypertrophy (Friedman Lingual Tonsil Scale).

Surgical technique

Preoperative planning

An awake flexible fiberoptic laryngoscopy should be performed to assess the tongue base. TBO should be suspected if the glottic inlet is only partially or minimally visible; this is caused by tongue base deflection of the epiglottis in a retrograde fashion over the larynx or frank obliteration of the larynx by the tongue base structures. Jaw-thrust maneuver will relieve glossoptosis but will have minimal effect on a hypertrophic LT. Anterior tongue extension (tongue pull) will roll the LT anterosuperiorly and relieve obstruction but will have minimal effect on reducing glossoptosis. Performing these 2 maneuvers will help differentiate the cause of obstruction between these 2. If both components are contributing to obstruction, then a combination of the 2 maneuvers will successfully relieve the obstruction. These maneuvers should be repeated during DISE to confirm the obstructive site or sites.

Preparation and patient positioning

- Nasal intubation provides optimal exposure of tongue base.
- Patient should be supine with a shoulder roll in place.
- A single dose of Unasyn or clindamycin and an airway dose of dexamethasone (0.5 mg/kg up to 12 mg) are administered.
- Dental bite block or Jennings retractor is placed to retract the oral cavity.

- A soft suction catheter is passed through the bilateral nasal cavities to retract the soft palate.
- A 2-0 silk retraction suture is placed in the midline tongue and helps elevate and expose the tongue base.

Surgical approach

- Lingual tonsillectomy and/or tongue base excision is performed transorally with endoscopic assistance.
- For most cases, a 70° 4-mm endoscope will provide excellent visualization of the operative field.
- In patients with dysmorphic craniofacial features, limited mandible mobility, or micrognathia, a 120° scope with palate retractor is used.
- The operating surgeon should be at the head of bed; the assistant should be at the side of the patient.

Surgical procedure

A radiofrequency coblation device with integrated suction is used. The LT is ablated down to the tongue base mucosa, from the vallecula to the circumvallate papilla in the rostro-caudal dimension, and from the pharyngeal wall to wall in the lateral dimension. Completely remove one-half of the tonsil from midline laterally before proceeding to the contralateral side (Figs. 2–4).

To proceed with tongue base excision or posterior midline glossectomy (removal of tongue musculature), the LT must first be completely removed. The same radiofrequency device is used to ablate the tongue muscle. Starting in the midline, a trough of tongue parenchyma is carefully removed from the vallecula anteriorly to the circumvallate papilla. Inferiorly, the width of the trough should be no wider than the base of the epiglottis (~10–12 mm). As the ablation extends anterosuperiorly, the width and depth of the trough should gradually increase. The final shape of the excision is dictated by the dimensions of the tongue musculature and oropharynx. Generally, 10 to 15 mm of tongue muscle is removed at the midline (Fig. 5).

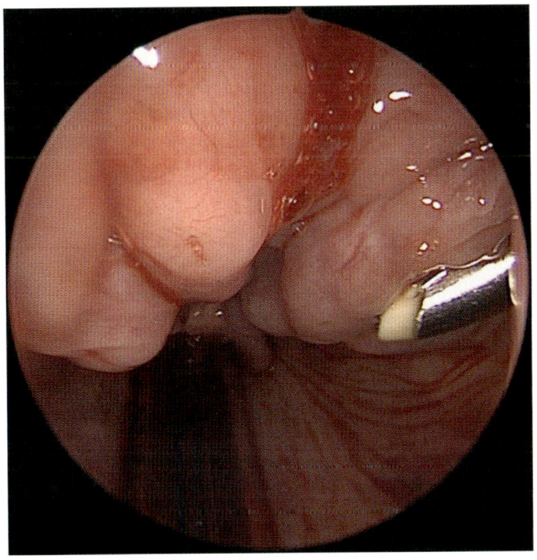

Fig. 2 Hypertrophied LT as visualized through a 70° endoscope. Nasal intubation provides excellent view of the entire tonsil. Note the relationship of the LT to the epiglottis.

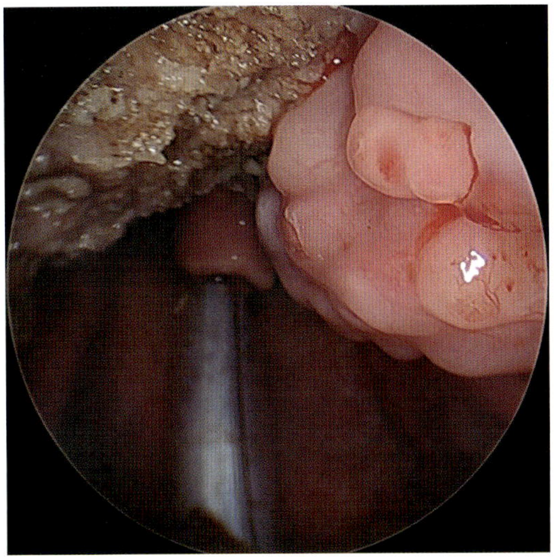

Fig. 3 Left side of LT completely removed.

Potential complications

1. Bleeding from the lingual artery: The paired arteries branch directly from the external carotid into the tongue musculature. They are located superficially at the base of the epiglottis on either side of midline and gradually course laterally and deep anteriorly. Transection of the main trunk or branches results in brisk and profuse bleeding. If bleeding cannot be controlled at the operative site, the vessel may require transarterial embolization or ligation via a transcervical open approach.

Bleeding from the inferior pole of the palatine tonsil fossa is more common with lingual tonsillectomy than tongue base (muscle) excision and is often due to a branch of the ascending pharyngeal or lingual arteries. It is similar in risk profile as when performing a standard palatine tonsillectomy.

2. Tongue paresthesia or dysesthesia caused by injury to the branches of the lingual nerve: This can be temporary or permanent.

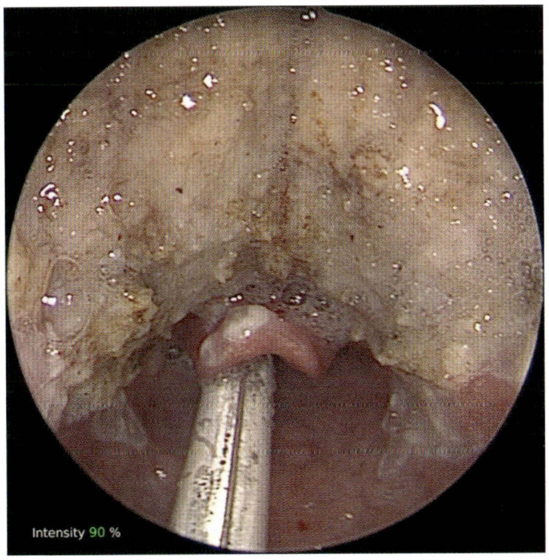

Fig. 4 LTs removed bilaterally.

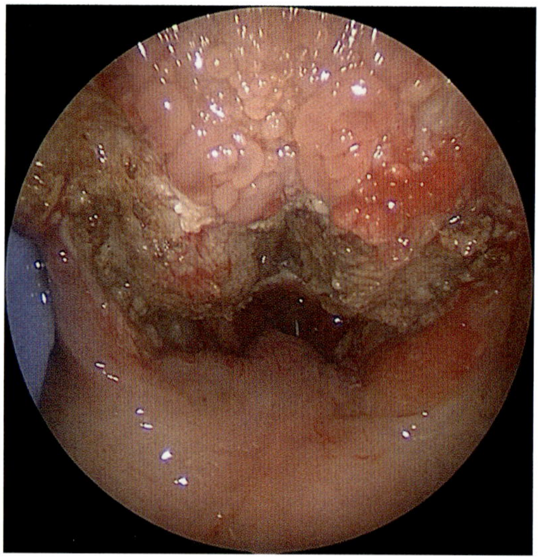

Fig. 5 Posterior midline glossectomy (tongue base excision).

3. Tongue paresis: Injury to the hypoglossal nerve (CN XII) can cause temporary or permanent weakness of the ipsilateral tongue.

Pearls and pitfalls

1. The lingual artery lies in close proximity to the base of epiglottis. Limiting the width of tongue base excision to the lateral dimension of the epiglottis at the vallecula minimizes the risk of injuring the lingual arteries or nerves.
2. In cases of markedly enlarged and fibrosed LTs, the tissue can be initially debulked with a monopolar diathermy device before finishing with the coblator. However, this requires retraction of the tissue with a second instrument, such as a forceps or clamp, and stabilization of the endoscope by the assistant. In craniofacial patients with trismus or narrow oral aperture, this may be technically difficult.
3. Always maintain movement of the coblation wand, because it can ablate tissue rapidly when stationary and result in inadvertent disruption of vessels.

Immediate postoperative care

- Apart from rare instances, the patient should be extubated in the operating room postoperatively.
- Intensive care unit admission for airway management is recommended in patients with moderate to severe OSA or those with comorbidities, such as hypotonia, genetic syndromes, obesity, and craniofacial anomalies.
- Additional doses of corticosteroids, but not antibiotics, are recommended.
- In the immediate perianesthetic period, persistent upper airway obstruction may be temporized with a nasopharyngeal airway or with the use of noninvasive positive pressure ventilation (NIPPV).

Rehabilitation and recovery

The postoperative recovery can last for 2 weeks. Postoperative pain is managed with nonsteroidal anti-inflammatory drugs and acetaminophen; opioids should be used sparingly (if at all) given its augmented deleterious effects on respiratory drive in patients with OSA. Odynophagia and otalgia are common. A soft diet is recommended. Secondary post-LT bleeding can occur, most commonly 5 to 7 days postoperatively.

Clinical results in the literature

In a 2016 study, DeMarcantonio and colleagues[5] assessed the safety and efficacy of lingual tonsillectomy in children with persistent OSA. They reported that 43.5% of these children had a syndromic diagnosis. The most common complications reported in their series included bleeding and presenting to emergency department (4.4%), poor oral intake (3.3%), and readmission (4.4%). In children with polysomnography data, the median Apnea Hypopnea Index (AHI) decreased from 8.5 to 3.8 events/h ($P = .022$). They concluded that lingual tonsillectomy is a safe and efficacious procedure in children with persistent OSA. Lingual tonsillectomy has a favorable postoperative course, but its effectiveness at curing residual OSA in the Down syndrome population has not been well established because these children tend to have significant glossoptosis, which results in persistent OSA that may warrant additional treatment.

In a recent systemic review and meta-analysis, Rivero and colleagues[6] evaluated the role of lingual tonsillectomy for pediatric persistent OSA. They analyzed 5 case series that met the study criteria and found lingual tonsillectomy to be a safe and effective surgery for persistent OSA in children with enlarged LT following Adenotonsillectomy (T&A). Lingual tonsillectomy reduces AHI (mean reduction 6.6/h), and the overall success rate (defined as postoperative OAHI $<$5/h) was 52%. These results indicate that, even though LT appears to be enlarged and recommending surgery seems to be logical, cure is not achieved in all cases because associated glossoptosis may play a role in partial response. Hence, a thorough evaluation of the causes of TBO should be undertaken before surgery to predict success and outcomes.

Summary

Lingual tonsillectomy and tongue base excision/ablation are effective surgical procedures in patients with TBO after adenotonsillectomy. Cine MRI of the upper airways and DISE is instrumental in confirming the site of obstruction. Improving the patency of the oropharyngeal and hypopharyngeal airway can result in resolution of persistent OSA in most patients; alternatively, this surgery may allow improved tolerance and use of NIPPV and/or reduction in the overall pressures required to treat persistent OSA in children.

References

1. Ishman SL, Chang KW, Kennedy AA. Techniques for evaluation and management of tongue-base obstruction in pediatric obstructive sleep apnea. Curr Opin Otolaryngol Head Neck Surg 2018;26(6):409–16.
2. Coutras SW, Limjuco A, Davis KE, et al. Sleep endoscopy findings in children with persistent obstructive sleep apnea after adenotonsillectomy. Int J Pediatr Otorhinolaryngol 2018;107:190–3.
3. Propst EJ, Amin R, Talwar N, et al. Midline posterior glossectomy and lingual tonsillectomy in obese and nonobese children with

down syndrome: biomarkers for success. Laryngoscope 2017;127(3): 757–63.
4. Abdel-Aziz M, Ibrahim N, Ahmed A, et al. Lingual tonsils hypertrophy; a cause of obstructive sleep apnea in children after adenotonsillectomy: operative problems and management. Int J Pediatr Otorhinolaryngol 2011;75(9):1127–31.
5. DeMarcantonio MA, Senser E, Meinzen-Derr J, et al. The safety and efficacy of pediatric lingual tonsillectomy. Int J Pediatr Otorhinolaryngol 2016;91:6–10.
6. Kang KT, Koltai PJ, Chee CH, et al. Lingual tonsillectomy for treatment of pediatric obstructive sleep apnea: a meta-analysis. JAMA Otolaryngol Head Neck Surg 2017;143(6):561–8.